Small Animal Dermatology

Editor

CHRISTINE L. CAIN

VETERINARY CLINICS OF NORTH AMERICA: SMALL ANIMAL PRACTICE

www.vetsmall.theclinics.com

January 2019 • Volume 49 • Number 1

ELSEVIER

1600 John F. Kennedy Boulevard • Suite 1800 • Philadelphia, Pennsylvania, 19103-2899
http://www.vetsmall.theclinics.com

VETERINARY CLINICS OF NORTH AMERICA: SMALL ANIMAL PRACTICE Volume 49, Number 1
January 2019 ISSN 0195-5616, ISBN-13: 978-0-323-67541-3

Editor: Colleen Dietzler
Developmental Editor: Meredith Madeira

Veterinary Clinics of North America: Small Animal Practice (ISSN 0195-5616) is published bimonthly by Elsevier Inc., 360 Park Avenue South, New York, NY 10010-1710. Months of issue are January, March, May, July, September, and November. Business and Editorial Offices: 1600 John F. Kennedy Blvd., Ste. 1800, Philadelphia, PA 19103-2899. Customer Service Office: 3251 Riverport Lane, Maryland Heights, MO 63043. Periodicals postage paid at New York, NY and additional mailing offices. Subscription prices are $338.00 per year (domestic individuals), $662.00 per year (domestic institutions), $100.00 per year (domestic students/residents), $451.00 per year (Canadian individuals), $823.00 per year (Canadian institutions), $474.00 per year (international individuals), $823.00 per year (international institutions), and $220.00 per year (international and Canadian students/residents). To receive student/resident rate, orders must be accompanied by name of affiliated institution, date of term, and the *signature* of program/residency coordinator on institution letterhead. Orders will be billed at individual rate until proof of status is received. Foreign air speed delivery is included in all *Clinics* subscription prices. All prices are subject to change without notice. **POSTMASTER:** Send address changes to *Veterinary Clinics of North America: Small Animal Practice*, Elsevier Health Sciences Division, Subscription Customer Service, 3251 Riverport Lane, Maryland Heights, MO 63043. Customer Service (orders, claims, online, change of address): Elsevier Periodicals Customer Service, Elsevier Health Sciences Division Subscription **Customer Service 3251 Riverport Lane Maryland Heights, MO 63043. Tel: 1-800-654-2452 (U.S. and Canada); 314-447-8871 (outside U.S. and Canada). Fax: 314-447-8029. E-mail: journalscustomerservice-usa@elsevier.com (for print support); journalsonlinesupport-usa@elsevier.com (for online support).**

Reprints. For copies of 100 or more of articles in this publication, please contact the Commercial Reprints Department, Elsevier Inc., 360 Park Avenue South, New York, NY 10010-1710. Tel.: 212-633-3874; Fax: 212-633-3820; E-mail: reprints@elsevier.com.

Veterinary Clinics of North America: Small Animal Practice is also published in Japanese by Inter Zoo Publishing Co., Ltd., Aoyama Crystal-Bldg 5F, 3-5-12 Kitaaoyama, Minato-ku, Tokyo 107-0061, Japan.

Veterinary Clinics of North America: Small Animal Practice is covered in *Current Contents/Agriculture, Biology and Environmental Sciences, Science Citation Index, ASCA, MEDLINE/PubMed (Index Medicus), Excerpta Medica, and BIOSIS.*

Contributors

EDITOR

CHRISTINE L. CAIN, DVM
Diplomate, American College of Veterinary Dermatology; Assistant Professor,
Dermatology, Department of Clinical Sciences and Advanced Medicine,
School of Veterinary Medicine, University of Pennsylvania, Philadelphia, Pennsylvania,
USA

AUTHORS

FRANE BANOVIC, DVM, PhD
Diplomate, European College of Veterinary Dermatology; Assistant Professor of
Dermatology, Department of Small Animal Medicine and Surgery, College of
Veterinary Medicine, University of Georgia, Athens, Georgia, USA

CHRISTINE L. CAIN, DVM
Diplomate, American College of Veterinary Dermatology; Assistant Professor,
Dermatology, Department of Clinical Sciences and Advanced Medicine,
School of Veterinary Medicine, University of Pennsylvania, Philadelphia, Pennsylvania,
USA

ELIZABETH A. MAULDIN, DVM
Diplomate, American College of Veterinary Pathologists; Diplomate, American College
of Veterinary Dermatology; Professor of Dermatopathology, University of Pennsylvania,
School of Veterinary Medicine, Philadelphia, Pennsylvania, USA

RALF S. MUELLER, DMV, MANZCVSc (Canine Medicine)
Diplomate, American College of Veterinary Dermatology; Fellow, Australian and
New Zealand College of Veterinary Scientists (Dermatology); Diplomate, European
College of Veterinary Dermatology; Professor of Veterinary Dermatology, Chief of
Allergology and Dermatology, Centre for Clinical Veterinary Medicine, Medizinische
Kleintierklinik, LMU Munich, Munich, Bavaria, Germany

CHIARA NOLI, DVM
Diplomate, European College of Veterinary Dermatology; Servizi Dermatologici Veterinari,
Peveragno, Cuneo, Italy

DIANE E. PREZIOSI, DVM
Diplomate, American College of Veterinary Dermatologists; Veterinary Specialists of
Alaska, Anchorage, Alaska, USA

KATHRYN A. ROOK, VMD
Diplomate, American College of Veterinary Dermatology; Clinical Assistant Professor
of Dermatology, Department of Clinical Sciences and Advanced Medicine, University
of Pennsylvania, School of Veterinary Medicine, Philadelphia, Pennsylvania, USA

DOMENICO SANTORO, DVM, MS, DrSc, PhD
Diplomate, American College of Veterinary Dermatology; Diplomate, European College of Veterinary Dermatology; Diplomate, American College of Veterinary Microbiologists (Bacteriology/Mycology and Immunology); Assistant Professor, Department of Small Animal Clinical Sciences, College of Veterinary Medicine, University of Florida, Gainesville, Florida, USA

JENNIFER SCHISSLER, DVM, MS
Diplomate, American College of Veterinary Dermatology; Assistant Professor, Dermatology and Otology, Colorado State University, James L. Voss Veterinary Teaching Hospital, Fort Collins, Colorado, USA

AMY K. SHUMAKER, DVM
Diplomate, American College of Veterinary Dermatology; Associate Veterinary Dermatologist, VCA South Shore (Weymouth) Animal Hospital, Weymouth, Massachusetts, USA

Contents

Allergen immunotherapy has been used for many years in dogs and cats and is the only specific treatment of atopic dermatitis that changes the patho-mechanisms of disease by stimulating allergen tolerance. Subcutaneous administration of allergens is the most commonly used administration route, typically in increasing concentrations (induction period) followed by long-term injection of allergen extract (maintenance therapy). Rush protocols with an abbreviated induction period have been reported and shown to be safe in dogs. More recently, oro-mucosal and intralymphatic administration of allergens has been evaluated in dogs. Approximately two-thirds of patients show good to excellent improvement of clinical signs.

Canine atopic dermatitis (AD) is one of the most common inflammatory skin diseases in dogs. The pathogenesis is complex and not completely understood. Many therapeutic options are available; however, because of cost, side effects, or a long lag phase, new compounds are constantly produced. This article provides a comprehensive review of the latest compounds for the treatment of canine AD. In addition, a brief review of new studies on conventional medications is provided. For a successful long-term therapeutic approach, it is important to considerate the status of the disease, as well as the patients' and their owners' needs.

Canine sterile pyogranulomatous dermatitis and panniculitis is an infrequently described syndrome. No autoantigen, or exogenous antigen, inflammatory stimulus has been identified. This syndrome is characterized by pyogranulomatous nodules, plaques, and ulcers of variable extent and severity. Prodromal and concurrent nonspecific clinical and hematologic signs of inflammation may occur. This waxing and waning condition is typically responsive to systemic immunomodulation. Lifelong therapy may be required to prevent relapse. Differential diagnoses include bacterial and fungal nodular dermatoses, neoplasia, and cutaneous reactive histiocytosis. Diagnosis is achieved via diagnostic exclusion of infectious causes and supportive histopathology findings.

As the spectrum of canine cutaneous lupus erythematosus (CLE) variants has expanded markedly in the recent 2 decades, veterinarians are encouraged to become familiar with the characteristic clinical features of CLE variants to permit early diagnosis and appropriate treatment. This article describes the signalment, clinical signs, treatment outcome, and laboratory and histopathology findings of 2 new canine CLE variants, generalized discoid lupus erythematosus and mucocutaneous lupus erythematosus.

Canine acute eosinophilic dermatitis with edema is an uncommon syndromic disorder in dogs with a unique clinical presentation. Most but not all dogs have a history of gastrointestinal upset preceding or concomitant with skin lesion onset. Affected dogs present with macular to generalized erythema that is most evident on the glabrous skin of the abdomen. Although the etiology is not known, an adverse drug reaction or a systemic type I hypersensitivity reaction may play a role. Some cases can be difficult to distinguish from canine sterile neutrophilic dermatosis due to overlapping clinical criteria and eosinophil degranulation in tissue section.

Canine perianal fistulas are painful sinus tracts and ulcers that spontaneously develop in the skin around the anus. Middle-aged German shepherd dogs are most commonly affected and may have a genetic susceptibility. Although the disease was once believed related to conformational factors and primarily managed surgically, an immune-mediated pathogenesis is now recognized. Long-term medical management with immunomodulatory agents has become standard of care for canine perianal fistulas. Perianal fistulas can be debilitating and have a negative impact on quality of life of dogs and owners. Accurate diagnosis and aggressive medical therapy are key to successful management of canine perianal fistulas.

Cutaneous lymphomas are divided into categories based on histologic evaluation of the skin and location of neoplastic lymphocytes. Epitheliotropic cutaneous lymphoma, also known as cutaneous T-cell lymphoma, is diagnosed when neoplastic lymphocytes show tropism for the epidermis and these cells infiltrate the epidermis and adnexae. In diagnosis of non-epitheliotropic cutaneous lymphoma, neoplastic lymphocytes are found mostly in the dermis and/or subcutis. Neoplastic cells are of either B-cell or T-cell origin. This article focuses on epitheliotropic cutaneous lymphomas and cutaneous lymphocytosis, which is considered a form of indolent lymphoma, in dogs and cats.

> Quality of life (QoL) is defined as "the degree to which an individual enjoys his or her life." In canine dermatology, 2 research groups have developed and validated questionnaires for QoL assessment in dogs with dermatologic conditions, the first being limited to canine atopic dermatitis, and the second one applicable to all skin conditions. A third group is working on the validation of a different QoL questionnaire coupled with a treatment success assessment tool. In general, there is an inverse correlation between QoL and pruritus.

> Feline pemphigus foliaceus is an uncommon skin disorder in cats but still the most common autoimmune skin disorder seen in this species. It is a crusting dermatosis involving the ears, head, paws, and ungual folds primarily. Although cytology is helpful in supporting a diagnosis, biopsy of pustules or crusts for histopathology is required for a definitive diagnosis. Therapy has evolved over the years as we have learned more about the different ways cats respond to drugs and as new drugs became available. Most cats will respond to proper therapy, although it may be needed long term for control.

> Acral lick dermatitis is a common, frustrating disease. It is characterized by incessant licking behavior resulting in raised, thickened, ulcerative plaques, most commonly affecting the lower extremities of dogs. Underlying primary diseases, such as allergic disorders (atopic dermatitis, food allergy, flea allergy), orthopedic or neurologic disorders, parasitic diseases (eg, demodicosis), infections (fungal, bacterial), neoplasia or psychogenic disorders (compulsive/obsessive-compulsive disorder), and perpetuating factors (especially secondary infections) drive the itch-lick cycle. Appropriately addressing the primary underlying disorder and secondary infections and addressing any possible behavioral component via behavioral modification and psychopharmacotherapeutics are vital for successful management of this disease.

VETERINARY CLINICS OF NORTH AMERICA: SMALL ANIMAL PRACTICE

SERIES OF RELATED INTEREST

Veterinary Clinics of North America: Exotic Animal Practice
https://www.vetexotic.theclinics.com/

THE CLINICS ARE NOW AVAILABLE ONLINE!
Access your subscription at:
www.theclinics.com

Preface

Small Animal Dermatology: Clinical Updates, Emerging Diseases, and Treatment Advances

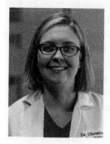

Christine L. Cain, DVM
Editor

Since publication of the last dermatology issue of *Veterinary Clinics of North America: Small Animal Practice* in 2013, considerable advances have been made in our understanding of the pathogenesis of dermatologic disease, particularly allergic skin disease. These advances have translated into new tools for the management of canine allergic dermatitis. The goals of this issue are to provide readers with a comprehensive review of therapeutic options for allergic dermatitis (with a focus on atopic dermatitis) as well as to review other dermatologic diseases that have been more recently described or are not thoroughly reviewed elsewhere in the veterinary medical literature. Each review provides practical guidelines for practitioners in disease recognition, diagnosis, and clinical management. My hope is that these articles will equip practitioners with the background knowledge necessary to tackle the clinical challenges presented by dermatologic diseases, and to highlight areas for further research and exploration within our exciting and ever-changing field.

Successful management of canine atopic dermatitis often requires a multimodal approach: improving the cutaneous barrier, managing secondary infections, and immunomodulation. The first article provides an update to clinicians on allergen-specific immunotherapy, including more recently implemented forms of immunotherapy in veterinary patients (sublingual immunotherapy and intralymphatic immunotherapy). The second article provides a comprehensive review of symptomatic management options for atopic dermatitis, with a focus on new and evolving therapies.

The authors of the next four articles review immune-mediated dermatoses that are emerging or have an incompletely elucidated pathogenesis. These articles review sterile inflammatory conditions: canine acute eosinophilic dermatitis with edema and

Vet Clin Small Anim 49 (2019) ix–x
https://doi.org/10.1016/j.cvsm.2018.09.001
0195-5616/19/© 2018 Published by Elsevier Inc.

sterile pyogranulomatous dermatitis and panniculitis, as well as canine perianal fistulas and two recently recognized forms of canine cutaneous lupus erythematosus.

Canine cutaneous epitheliotropic T-cell lymphoma is one of the most devastating conditions encountered in small animal dermatology and carries a poor prognosis. It can also be one of the most challenging conditions for practitioners to recognize given its clinical similarities to other dermatoses. The author of this article reviews the clinical presentation, diagnosis, prognosis, and treatment options for canine cutaneous epithelitropic T-cell lymphoma as well as two rare forms of cutaneous lymphoma: feline cutaneous epitheliotropic lymphoma and cutaneous lymphocytosis.

The importance of quality of life in pets with dermatologic disease as well as the owners of pets with dermatologic disease cannot be overstated. Many skin conditions, including several of those highlighted in this issue, are chronic, incurable, and associated with the need for lifelong or labor-intensive management. One article in this issue details the development and validation of tools for the assessment of quality of life in dogs and cats with dermatologic disease. These tools will allow the evaluation of quality of life (of patients and pet owners) as an additional metric for determining treatment success in clinical trials, which guide our evidence-based practice of veterinary dermatology.

Two articles review common conditions in small animal dermatology. One article emphasizes a practical approach to clinical recognition, diagnosis (including tips for optimal skin biopsy technique), and management of feline pemphigus foliaceus, the most common autoimmune dermatosis of cats. In another article, the author provides a useful algorithm for approaching the diagnostic workup and management of patients with acral lick dermatitis. Like many other chronic skin conditions, successful management requires the clinician to recognize and effectively address multiple primary and perpetuating factors.

It was a privilege serving as guest editor of this issue. I would like to sincerely thank my colleagues for their hard work and dedication in lending their expertise to these articles.

Christine L. Cain, DVM
Department of Clinical Sciences and
Advanced Medicine
School of Veterinary Medicine
University of Pennsylvania
3900 Delancey Street
Philadelphia, PA 19104, USA

E-mail address:
ccain@vet.upenn.edu

Update on Allergen Immunotherapy

Ralf S. Mueller, DMV

KEYWORDS

- Allergen specific • Desensitization • Hyposensitization • Feline • Canine
- Intralymphatic

KEY POINTS

- Allergen immunotherapy is the only specific therapy for atopic dermatitis in dogs and cats.
- Selection of allergens should be based on clinical history of the animal in conjunction with positive reactions on intradermal or serum testing.
- To optimize success, the protocol should be individualized to each patient; when adapting the dose and/or frequency during the treatment, most animals show a good to excellent response.
- Adverse effects include increased pruritus and very rarely anaphylactic reactions.
- Subcutaneous, intralymphatic, and oro-mucosal administration routes have been reported; the subcutaneous route is most frequently used.

INTRODUCTION

Allergen immunotherapy (AIT) is the only treatment of atopic dermatitis that is able to change the pathogenic mechanisms of the disease. By injecting relevant allergens, AIT aims at initiating an immune response that leads to activation of regulatory T cells and immunosuppressive cytokines with a subsequent improvement of clinical signs. In the past, the term *allergen-specific immunotherapy* was used; but as AIT by definition contains specific allergens, AIT is as accurate and avoids stating the obvious. AIT has been used successfully in several animal species but is most commonly used in dogs. Data in cats are more limited. Initially, AIT was administered subcutaneously; but intralymphatic and sublingual or oral immunotherapy protocols have also been described.

Disclosure Statement: In the last 5 years, R.S. Mueller has received support from Artu Biologicals and Heska Corporation for studies evaluating immunotherapy and serum testing for identification of allergens involved in canine atopic dermatitis, respectively.
Centre for Clinical Veterinary Medicine, Medizinische Kleintierklinik, LMU Munich, Veterinaerstr. 13, Munich 80539, Bavaria, Germany
E-mail address: R.Mueller@lmu.de

SELECTION OF ALLERGENS FOR ALLERGEN IMMUNOTHERAPY

For many years, intradermal testing was the gold standard for the identification of offending allergens in animals with atopic dermatitis. Today serum tests for allergen-specific immunoglobulin E (IgE) are also used, and the success rate of AIT seems to be the same when allergens are chosen based on skin testing compared with serum testing.[1] Interassay and intraassay variability of serum testing has been evaluated in several studies, some of which showed a high reproducibility[2]; in others the reproducibility was much lower,[3] emphasizing the need for independent evaluation of a testing method before it can be recommended. As healthy dogs show numerous positive reactions on both skin and serum tests,[4,5] allergens should be chosen not only based on test results but also on clinical history. For example, if in a temperate climate an atopic dog shows severe pruritus all year round yet only has a strong reaction to birch pollen, this would not explain its clinical signs. Similarly, in a dog that exhibits clinical signs only in spring or summer and shows a strong positive reaction to house dust mites, it is unlikely the clinical signs are due to dust mites. Positive skin test or serum test results indicate sensitization against an allergen with subsequent IgE production, not necessarily clinically relevant hypersensitivity. Consequently, skin or serum test results are not suitable to make a diagnosis of environmental allergies in any species because of those false-positive reactions and should only be used with the aim to identify allergens suitable for AIT in animals that are diagnosed with atopic dermatitis based on history, clinical examination, and having ruled out differential diagnoses. Thus, pros and cons of AIT need to be discussed with the owners and AIT chosen as desired therapy before performing those tests. Subsequently, the results of either intradermal testing or testing for allergen-specific IgE should be interpreted in light of the clinical history of that particular patient; the allergens included in the treatment solution should be chosen based on this history.

MECHANISM OF ACTION

Most available information about the mechanism of action of AIT derives from studies with dogs and parallels what is seen in humans (**Box 1**). An increase in so-called blocking IgG antibodies was described in dogs undergoing immunotherapy[6,7]; but an actual binding and, thus, inactivation of offending allergens by those antibodies have not been demonstrated as of yet; it is not known whether production of those allergen-specific antibodies during AIT is correlated to a good clinical response. An increase in FoxP3+ regulatory T cells and IL-10 and a decrease in allergen-specific IgE have been associated with successful immunotherapy in one study.[8] In cats with experimental asthma that underwent rush immunotherapy (RIT) with CpG

Box 1
Mechanisms of action of allergen immunotherapy in dogs and humans

- IgG4 ↑
- FoxP3+ CD4+ Treg ↑
- IL-10 ↑
- IL-4 ↓
- IgE ↓

Abbreviations: IgG4, immunoglobulin G4; IL, interleukin; Treg, regulatory T cell.

oligodeoxynucleotides, the percentage of eosinophils in the bronchoalveolar lavage fluid (BALF) decreased significantly with immunotherapy; but the number of regulatory T cells in the peripheral blood and the concentration of IL-10 or interferon-gamma in the BALF did not change.[9]

SUBCUTANEOUS ALLERGEN IMMUNOTHERAPY

Traditionally, allergens in AIT of canine atopic dermatitis (as in other species) are injected subcutaneously during the induction period in gradually increasing volume and concentration over a few weeks to a few months depending on the protocol.[10] Thereafter maintenance therapy is administered with the same amount of allergen extract every few weeks to once monthly for a period of several years. However, most dermatologists agree that the amount of allergen and the frequency of injections have to be adjusted to individual patients. If a dog shows increased pruritus directly after the injection, that then subsides again a few days later, the dose should be reduced at the next injection. If the pruritus improves after the injections but then increases again some time before the next allergen administration, a shorter interval between injections is advisable. The final response should not be evaluated until 12 months after beginning AIT. Owners need to be made aware before choosing immunotherapy that it may take 1 year until maximal improvement has been achieved.

Patients on immunotherapy may need additional antipruritic medication during the first months of treatment. Essential fatty acids, antihistamines, lokivetmab, and shampoo therapy are unlikely to interfere with tolerance induction. However, the author prefers not to use glucocorticoids, cyclosporine, and oclacitinib as long-term therapy during the first year of AIT but rather as short treatment courses as needed.

Many studies evaluating subcutaneous AIT (SCIT) show an excellent response or a good improvement in approximately two-thirds of the dogs, independent of age, sex, breed, type of allergen, perennial or seasonal clinical signs, and high- or low-dose protocols (**Table 1**).[1] The few studies evaluating RIT, oro-mucosal immunotherapy (OIT), and intralymphatic immunotherapy (ILIT) reported similar success rates.[11–13] However, most studies included a small number of dogs and were case studies[1]; only a few studies were randomized and double blinded.[12,14,15] Thus, the results need to be interpreted with caution; more studies are needed to determine factors optimizing treatment outcomes. In addition, dose-finding studies were performed only, rarely, in dogs; their results have not been conclusive.[1,15,16]

Table 1		
Success rate of canine allergen immunotherapy in various studies		
Study Reference	Success Rate (% Good to Excellent Responders)	Number of Dogs Included
Keppel et al,[8] 2008	51	53
Mueller & Bettenay,[17] 1996	58	146
Nuttall et al,[18] 1998	22[a]	186
Schnabl et al,[16] 2006	64	117
Scott et al,[19] 1993	60	144
Zur et al,[20] 2002	52	169

[a] Most studies evaluated responses as excellent, good, mild/moderate, and poor; this particular study only graded responses as good, partial, or none; 22% showed a good and 39% a partial response.

RUSH IMMUNOTHERAPY

With subcutaneous RIT, the induction period of several weeks to months is abbreviated to 1 day and injections are given hourly. Dogs are continuously monitored clinically in a hospital setting. In human medicine, RIT is performed to achieve a more rapid improvement, particularly in patients with venom hypersensitivities, but is associated with a high rate of anaphylactoid reactions. In dogs, RIT is well tolerated and has mainly been associated with increased pruritus; more severe reactions have been extremely rare.[12,21] The protocol in dogs includes a recommendation of an antihistamine administration 1 or 2 hours before the injection of the allergen extract. In a double-blinded study, the maximum improvement in clinical signs was reached after 6.8 months with RIT compared with 9.2 months with classic immunotherapy; however, in this study the difference failed to reach statistical significance.[12] RIT with alum-precipitated allergens has been reported with similar safety and success rates as RIT with aqueous allergens.[22] RIT has also been reported in 4 cats,[23] but this number is too small to make any conclusions about safety; efficacy was not reported in this case series.

ORO-MUCOSAL IMMUNOTHERAPY

Oral immunotherapy has been available in some countries for several years. In humans with sublingual immunotherapy (SLIT), small amounts of allergens are administered and kept under the tongue for several minutes without swallowing; in oral immunotherapy, allergens are swallowed after oral administration. In dogs, a small amount of extract is applied between the lips and gums once to twice daily. Consequently, in animals, OIT is probably the better term. Improvement of clinical signs and a decrease in allergen-specific IgE were reported in a small number of dogs with this type of AIT.[13] A larger clinical study a few years ago showed a reasonable success rate comparable with that seen with SCIT.[24] In addition, dogs improved on OIT that had previously failed to improve on SCIT. Unfortunately, this study is not published. Further scientific studies are needed to evaluate optimal treatment protocols for this treatment option.

INTRALYMPHATIC IMMUNOTHERAPY

In humans, ILIT is associated with a prolonged improvement after 3 monthly injections and was reported to be safer and better tolerated than SCIT.[25,26] In dogs, several studies have evaluated ILIT and reported it a safe treatment alternative to SCIT or OIT.[11,27,28] A smaller amount of allergen extract (typically 0.1 mL) is injected in the submandibular or popliteal lymph node monthly. Based on published data, prolonged improvement is only seen in a small number of dogs; most patients will need continuous intralymphatic or subcutaneous injections, especially when aqueous allergens are used.[27] The author has seen some dogs improve on ILIT that previously failed to improve on SCIT. Short- and midterm adverse effects seem to be very rare.[11,27,28] Long-term adverse effects of ILIT are not known, and further studies about long-term safety are particularly needed with alum-precipitated extracts.

FELINE ALLERGEN IMMUNOTHERAPY

Atopic dermatitis in cats is not well defined. There is evidence for causal involvement of allergens in cats with noninflammatory alopecia, severe head and neck pruritus, lesions of the eosinophilic granuloma complex, miliary dermatitis, and feline asthma.[9,29] In cats with skin disease, few studies are published evaluating AIT; almost all of them evaluated SCIT in a small number of cats.[1,29–31] All of those studies showed success rates similar to what is seen in dogs with atopic dermatitis. One study reported successful RIT in 4 cats.[23] No studies have been published evaluating ILIT or SLIT in cats. More information is published about the treatment of cats with asthma sensitized to various allergens in a laboratory setting.[32] Successful RIT with a decrease in eosinophil numbers in bronchoalveolar lavage has been reported even when the allergen used in the extract was either not the allergen the cats were sensitized to or not the only allergen the cats were sensitized to.[33] When bacterial oligodeoxynucleotides were used as an adjuvant to RIT in those cats with experimental asthma, eosinophilic airway inflammation was also significantly alleviated.[9]

ADVERSE EFFECTS OF IMMUNOTHERAPY

Increased pruritus after allergen administration is the most common adverse effect seen with subcutaneous immunotherapy.[1] In many cases, this can be alleviated by decreasing the volume of allergen extract injected. Other animals may benefit from the administration of an antihistamine 2 hours before allergen injection. In some cases, this may be due to adjuvants; in a double-blinded study 3 of 27 dogs treated with alum-precipitate allergens and 2 of 24 dogs treated with an alum-containing placebo showed generalized pruritus.[14] Localized injection reactions may rarely be seen.[1] In a small number of patients (<1%), systemic reactions may occur and include anxiety, depression, diarrhea, hyperactivity, sleepiness, urticaria/angioedema, vomiting, weakness, and very rarely collapse and anaphylaxis.[1] For milder adverse effects, glucocorticoids or antihistamines may be administered; however, in patients with anaphylaxis, intravenous epinephrine is the treatment of choice.

SUMMARY

AIT is a good treatment option for environmental allergy in dogs and cats. It is the only specific therapy and the only treatment reported to change the patho-mechanisms of the disease. Subcutaneous immunotherapy combines a satisfactory success rate with a good safety profile. Anaphylactic reactions are rarely seen in animals. In addition to the subcutaneous administration of allergens, more recent routes of administration, such as intralymphatic and OIT, have been described. Pilot studies with different adjuvants, such as bacterial oligodeoxynucleotides,[9,34,35] pullulan,[36] or mannan,[37] have been published; their use may further increase safety and efficacy. The first trials have reported the use of recombinant allergens.[38] However, as most of the published studies are case series with often rather small numbers of animals included, more and larger randomized studies of immunotherapy are needed in a clinical setting to provide guidance on the optimal selection of allergens, adjuvants, dosing, success rate, and adverse effects of the various protocols of immunotherapy in dogs and cats.

REFERENCES

1. Loewenstein C, Mueller RS. A review of allergen-specific immunotherapy in human and veterinary medicine. Vet Dermatol 2009;20:84–98.
2. Thom N, Favrot C, Failing K, et al. Intra- and interlaboratory variability of allergen-specific IgE levels in atopic dogs in three different laboratories using the Fc-epsilon receptor testing. Vet Immunol Immunopathol 2010;133:183–9.
3. Patterson AP, Schaeffer DJ, Campbell KL. Reproducibility of a commercial in vitro allergen-specific assay for immunoglobulin E in dogs. Vet Rec 2005;157:81–5.

4. Mueller RS, Fieseler KV, Rosychuk RA, et al. Intradermal testing with the storage mite *Tyrophagus putrescentiae* in normal dogs and dogs with atopic dermatitis in Colorado. Vet Dermatol 2005;16:27–31.
5. Lian TM, Halliwell RE. Allergen-specific IgE and IgGd antibodies in atopic and normal dogs. Vet Immunol Immunopathol 1998;66:203–23.
6. Hou CC, Griffin CE, Hill PB. Dermatophagoides farinae-specific IgG responses in atopic dogs undergoing allergen-specific immunotherapy with aqueous vaccines. Vet Dermatol 2008;19:215–20.
7. Hites MJ, Kleinbeck ML, Loker JL, et al. Effect of immunotherapy on the serum concentrations of allergen-specific IgG antibodies in dog sera. Vet Immunol Immunopathol 1989;22:39–51.
8. Keppel KE, Campbell KL, Zuckermann FA, et al. Quantitation of canine regulatory T cell populations, serum interleukin-10 and allergen-specific IgE concentrations in healthy control dogs and canine atopic dermatitis patients receiving allergen-specific immunotherapy. Vet Immunol Immunopathol 2008;123:337–44.
9. Reinero CR, Cohn LA, Delgado C, et al. Adjuvanted rush immunotherapy using CpG oligodeoxynucleotides in experimental feline allergic asthma. Vet Immunol Immunopathol 2008;121:241–50.
10. Griffin CE, Hillier A. The ACVD task force on canine atopic dermatitis (XXIV): allergen-specific immunotherapy. Vet Immunol Immunopathol 2001;81:363–83.
11. Timm K, Mueller RS, Nett-Mettler CS. Long term effects of intralymphatic immunotherapy (ILIT) in canine atopic dermatitis. Vet Dermatol 2018;29:123–30.
12. Mueller RS, Fieseler KV, Zabel S, et al. Conventional and rush immunotherapy in canine atopic dermatitis. In: Hillier A, Foster AP, Kwochka KW, editors. Advances in veterinary dermatology V. Oxford (England): Blackwell Publishing; 2005. p. 60–9.
13. DeBoer DJ, Verbrugge M, Morris M. Clinical and immunological responses of dust mite sensitive, atopic dogs to treatment with sublingual immunotherapy (SLIT). Vet Dermatol 2016;27:82–87e23.
14. Willemse A, Van den Brom WE, Rijnberk A. Effect of hyposensitization on atopic dermatitis in dogs. J Am Vet Med Assoc 1984;184:1277–80.
15. Colombo S, Hill PB, Shaw DJ, et al. Effectiveness of low dose immunotherapy in the treatment of canine atopic dermatitis: a prospective, double-blinded, clinical study. Vet Dermatol 2005;16:162–70.
16. Schnabl B, Bettenay SV, Dow K, et al. Results of allergen-specific immunotherapy in 117 dogs with atopic dermatitis. Vet Rec 2006;158:81–5.
17. Mueller RS, Bettenay SV. Long-term immunotherapy of 146 dogs with atopic dermatitis - a retrospective study. Aust Vet Pract 1996;26:128.
18. Nuttall TJ, Thoday KL, van den Broek AH, et al. Retrospective survey of allergen immunotherapy in canine atopy. Vet Rec 1998;143:139–42.
19. Scott KV, White SD, Rosychuk RAW. A retrospective study of hyposensitization in atopic dogs in a flea scarce environment. In: Ihrke PJ, Mason IS, White SD, editors. Advances in veterinary dermatology. Oxford (England): Pergamon Press; 1993. p. 79–87.
20. Zur G, White SD, Ihrke PJ, et al. Canine atopic dermatitis: a retrospective study of 169 cases examined at the University of California, Davis, 1992-1998. Part II. Response to hyposensitization. Vet Dermatol 2002;13:103–11.
21. Mueller RS, Bettenay SV. Evaluation of the safety of an abbreviated course of injections of allergen extracts (rush immunotherapy) for the treatment of dogs with atopic dermatitis. Am J Vet Res 2001;62:307–10.

22. Hobi S, Mueller RS. Efficacy and safety of rush immunotherapy with alum-precipitated allergens in canine atopic dermatitis. Tierarztl Prax Ausg K Kleintiere Heimtiere 2014;42:167–73.
23. Trimmer AM, Griffin CE, Boord MJ, et al. Rush allergen specific immunotherapy protocol in feline atopic dermatitis: a pilot study of four cats. Vet Dermatol 2005;16:324–9.
24. DeBoer D, Morris M. Multicentre open trial demonstrates efficacy of sublingual immunotherapy in canine atopic dermatitis (abstract). Vet Dermatol 2012;23:65.
25. Senti G, Crameri R, Kuster D, et al. Intralymphatic immunotherapy for cat allergy induces tolerance after only 3 injections. J Allergy Clin Immunol 2012;129:1290–6.
26. Hylander T, Larsson O, Petersson-Westin U, et al. Intralymphatic immunotherapy of pollen-induced rhinoconjunctivitis: a double-blind placebo-controlled trial. Respir Res 2016;17:10.
27. Hatzmann K, Mueller RS. Practicability and safety of intralymphatic allergen-specific immunotherapy in dogs with atopic dermatitis. Annual Congress of the European Society of Veterinary Dermatology. Bruxelles: Veterinary Dermatology, 2011;463–4.
28. Fischer N, Rostaher A, Favrot C. Intralymphatic immunotherapy: an effective and safe alternative route for canine atopic dermatitis. Schweiz Arch Tierheilkd 2016;158:646–52.
29. Ravens PA, Xu BJ, Vogelnest LJ. Feline atopic dermatitis: a retrospective study of 45 cases (2001-2012). Vet Dermatol 2014;25:95–102.
30. Prost C. Atopy in the cat: 28 cases. Proceedings of the Second World Congress of Veterinary Dermatology, Montreal, Canada, 1992; p. 87.
31. Bettenay SV. Response to hyposensitization in 29 atopic cats. In: Kwochka KW, Willemse A, von Tscharner C, editors. Advances in veterinary dermatology. Oxford (England): Butterworth/Heinemann; 1998. p. 517–8.
32. Norris Reinero CR, Decile KC, Berghaus RD, et al. An experimental model of allergic asthma in cats sensitized to house dust mite or bermuda grass allergen. Int Arch Allergy Immunol 2004;135:117–31.
33. Reinero C, Lee-Fowler T, Chang CH, et al. Beneficial cross-protection of allergen-specific immunotherapy on airway eosinophilia using unrelated or a partial repertoire of allergen(s) implicated in experimental feline asthma. Vet J 2012;192:412–6.
34. Rostaher A, Fuchs S, Weber K, et al. Immunomodulatory effects of CPG oligodeoxynucleotides delivered by gelatine nanoparticles in the treatment of canine atopic dermatitis – a pilot study. Vet Dermatol 2013;24:494–500.
35. Mueller RS, Veir J, Fieseler KV, et al. Use of immunostimulatory liposome-nucleic acid complexes in allergen-specific immunotherapy of dogs with refractory atopic dermatitis - a pilot study. Vet Dermatol 2005;16:61–8.
36. Kawano K, Mizuno T. A pilot study of the effect of pullulan-conjugated Der f 2 allergen-specific immunotherapy on canine atopic dermatitis. Vet Dermatol 2017;28:583-e141.
37. Soria I, Alvarez J, Manzano AI, et al. Mite allergoids coupled to nonoxidized mannan from Saccharomyces cerevisae efficiently target canine dendritic cells for novel allergy immunotherapy in veterinary medicine. Vet Immunol Immunopathol 2017;190:65–72.
38. Olivry T, Paps JS, Dunston SM. Proof of concept of the preventive efficacy of high-dose recombinant mono-allergen immunotherapy in atopic dogs sensitized to the Dermatophagoides farinae allergen Der f 2. Vet Dermatol 2017;28:183-e140.

Therapies in Canine Atopic Dermatitis: An Update

Domenico Santoro, DVM, MS, DrSc, PhD

KEYWORDS

• Atopic dermatitis • Dog • Therapy • Review

KEY POINTS

• Canine atopic dermatitis is a multifaceted chronic disease requiring a tailored therapeutic approach.
• New therapies have been designed for canine atopic dermatitis.
• Alternative and topical therapies are fundamental in the management of canine atopic dermatitis.
• Future therapies may include more biologics and more tailored treatments based on the individual clinical presentation.

INTRODUCTION

Atopic dermatitis (AD) is one of the most common cutaneous inflammatory and pruritic diseases in dogs. AD is a genetically predisposed inflammatory and pruritic skin disease associated with well-defined clinical signs and immunoglobulin (Ig)E directed against environmental allergens.[1] Atopiclike dermatitis (ADL) is a disease characterized by the same clinical signs of AD in absence of demonstrable IgE.[1] The major difference between these 2 entities resides in the impossibility to demonstrate IgE in ADL, making it impossible to formulate an allergen-specific immunotherapy (ASIT).[1] The true incidence of ADL is unknown, and the therapeutic response to the common therapies for AD is also unknown. In one unpublished study performed in France by Prelaud and Cochet-Faivre,[2] 25.6% of dogs enrolled were diagnosed with ADL. A similar percentage (14.6%) was present in a more recent study in the United States.[3] A breed predisposition for English bulldogs was also suspected in one of these studies.[2] In addition, the efficacy of cyclosporine (CsA) for such patients is controversial. In the first study, a lower efficacy rate was seen in ADL compared with AD dogs (50% vs 92%)[2]; although in other studies, CsA has been shown to be effective in ADL dogs.[3,4] The effect of more recent drugs on ADL is unknown. The difficulty to treat AD/

Disclosure Statement: The author has nothing to disclose.
Department of Small Animal Clinical Sciences, College of Veterinary Medicine, University of Florida, 2015 Southwest 16th Avenue, Gainesville, FL 32610, USA
E-mail address: dsantoro@ufl.edu

ADL dogs resides also in the well-known diversity in clinical presentation and response to treatments within the 2 AD entities. Because of this enormous diversity, canine AD has been recently suggested to be classified as a syndrome more than a well-defined single cutaneous inflammatory entity, as proposed in human AD.[5]

CANINE ATOPIC DERMATITIS: CLINICAL AND PATHOGENETIC SYNOPSIS

AD is extremely common in dogs, affecting between 3% and 15% of the canine population or up to 58% of dogs affected by skin diseases.[6–8] The age of onset typically spans between 6 months and 6 years; however, more than 70% of AD dogs develop clinical signs between 1 and 3 years of age. Many breeds have been associated with AD, with terriers, retrievers, and brachycephalic dogs most commonly affected.[9–11]

Clinically, canine AD is characterized by chronic skin inflammation, pruritus, and recurrent skin infections. The most common clinical signs include generalized pruritus (seasonal, nonseasonal, or nonseasonal with seasonal worsening), erythema, papules, pustules, crusts, and excoriations.[12] Head (perioral, periocular, and ears), flexor aspect of elbows, carpal and tarsal joints, paws (digits, claws, and interdigital aspects), ventral abdomen, perineum, and ventral tail are most commonly affected.[12] However, few exceptions have been reported in West Highland white terriers, sharpeis, and German shepherds.[13] The diagnosis of canine AD is based on characteristic clinical signs and by excluding other pruritic diseases (eg, food allergy, demodicosis, scabies).[12]

The pathogenesis of AD is very complex and not completely elucidated. Both genetic and environmental factors are involved in the development of the clinical disease, with both types I and IV hypersensitivity reactions demonstrated. Classically, the first step involved in the development of AD is a sensitization to environmental allergens (eg, house dust mites) penetrating through the skin (mainly) able to lead to recruitment and activation of resident inflammatory cells and degranulation of mast cells via binding to IgE. On activation, multiple inflammatory mediators, including cytokines (specifically type 2 and proinflammatory) and chemokines are secreted, determining the course of the disease. With the chronicity of the lesions, a type 1 inflammatory response predominates. Last, a defect in the epidermal barrier is associated to a higher penetration of allergens through the skin and exacerbation of the inflammatory response. However, if such defect is primary or secondary is still controversial. Other major exacerbating factors include bacterial (Staphylococcus pseudintermedius) and fungal (Malassezia pachydermatis) infections along with psychogenic and environmental (eg, humidity) factors. Very recently, a series of review articles has been published. The series represents an extensive review on the current knowledge on the pathogenesis of canine AD.[14–20] Thus, for more in-depth information, the author refers the reader to such review articles.

Due to the diversity of the phenomena involved in the pathogenesis of canine AD and the variety of clinical presentations, a more rational and tailored therapeutic approach is required for each patient.[21,22] Such therapeutic options should be customized for each atopic dog, keeping in consideration the needs of each dog (eg, amount of drugs, side effects, severity of the clinical signs, easy administration of treatments) and the dog's owners (eg, financial circumstances, expectations, quality of life, time).

TREATMENT OVERVIEW

The treatment of canine AD is mainly centered on 4 factors: time (chronic vs acute lesions), presence of pruritus, inflammation, and infections. The chronicity of the lesions and their severity will determine the choice of short-term (eg, flare) versus long-term medications, keeping in mind side effects, efficacy, and costs. Finally, cutaneous infections, bacterial and/or fungal, are major exacerbators, and as such need to be properly treated. Topical and systemic options are commercially available to treat AD. For the purpose of this review, only therapies that are available for dogs are discussed in depth. Finally, a discussion on ASIT, injectable or sublingual, is beyond the scope of this review.

TOPICAL THERAPIES

Recently, 2 documents highlighting the guidelines for the treatment of canine AD have shown that the improvement of the skin, and coat hygiene and care is fundamental in treating atopic dogs.[21,22] The skin care can be achieved in several ways by using different products with the goal of moisturizing the skin, reducing the inflammatory and/or pruritic response, and repairing the skin barrier.

MOISTURIZERS

Moisturizers (emollients and/or humectants) have multiple functions. The most important action is increasing the amount of water in the skin by reducing the transepidermal water loss (TEWL) via blocking agents (ie, oils) or using hygroscopic molecules. These latter act as occlusive agents and attract water from the environment and/or from the dermis/subcutaneous tissues (eg, oatmeal). The increase of hydration alone is able to significantly reduce the pruritus and the need of antipruritic drugs; weekly Allermyl shampoo (containing lipids, complex sugars, and antiseptics) for 3 to 4 weeks significantly decreases pruritus and lesional score in most dogs.[23,24]

ANTI-INFLAMMATORY/ANTIPRURITIC

The most important topical anti-inflammatory drugs include glucocorticoids (GCs) and calcineurin inhibitors (CIs); however, antihistamines and local anesthetics have been used in dogs with some success.

GCs are extremely potent and versatile compounds that can be used either systemically or topically. They are generally associated to a significant reduction in both inflammation and pruritus. Their mechanism of action is very broad, complex, and not completely understood. In allergic diseases, they seem to interfere with proinflammatory and pruritogenic mediators, inflammatory cell migration and function, and with inflammation-associated nerve hypersensitivity.[25]

Topical GCs have been largely used during the past decades for the reduced presence of systemic side effects (eg, polyuria, polydipsia, polyphagia, urinary tract infections, and muscle wasting) compared with oral GCs; however, cutaneous atrophy, comedones, and calcinosis cutis are potential side effects for some topical GCs. Based on their chemical structure, topical GCs can be divided into "old" and "new" generation. To the former belong compounds like hydrocortisone, prednisolone, triamcinolone acetonide, betamethasone, and dexamethasone. The new generation includes diester topical GCs, like mometasone furoate, hydrocortisone aceponate, and prednicarbate. These latter are metabolized in situ into inactive molecules, dramatically reducing the presence of systemic side effects.

Triamcinolone acetonide (0.015%, Genesis; Virbac, Fort Worth, TX) spray is the only "old" GC that has been shown to be highly efficacious in the treatment of canine AD. In a multicenter, randomized, double-blinded, placebo/vehicle-controlled clinical trial (RDBPCT),[26] triamcinolone acetonide spray was applied to allergic dogs for 4 weeks at tapered frequency. At the end of the study, a significant improvement in pruritus, clinical signs, and overall assessment was present when compared with vehicle in absence of clinical and minor hematological adverse effects (slightly lower total leukocyte, lymphocyte, and eosinophil counts after treatment).

Similar response has been documented for hydrocortisone aceponate (0.0584%, Cortavance; Virbac), a "new" GC, through few RDBPCTs trials in Europe and Korea.[27-30] In the first clinical trial,[27] Cortavance was administered to dogs with mild AD for 70 days at tapered frequency. After 28 days of treatment, 73.0% and 46.6% of dogs achieved a reduction of $\geq$50% in clinical score and pruritus, respectively. These results were confirmed by a second study[28] comparing the efficacy of daily Cortavance with cyclosporine over 84 days.[27] This study showed the clinical equivalence between Cortavance and CsA in absence of clinical, hematological, or hormonal abnormalities.[26,27] Similarly, a third study[29] using Cortavance for 14 days showed a significant decrease in clinical signs, pruritus, and TEWL in absence of side effects, suggesting a positive effect of hydrocortisone aceponate on skin barrier function. Another RDBPCT[30] showed promising effects of Cortavance as prophylactic treatment (twice weekly), able to prolong the remission time in atopic dogs. Finally, more recently, the immunologic effects of Cortavance have also been assessed in 2 other studies performed in the United States[31] and Japan.[32] In the first study,[31] the investigators showed that once-daily Cortavance spray for 14 days is able to interfere with intradermal testing (IDT) in dogs, and a minimum of 2 weeks is necessary to avoid such effect on IDT. In addition, this was the first study showing that Cortavance may be able to induce, histologically, a significant decrease in dermal thickness that may be present. In addition, Cortavance may also induce, when used daily for 3 weeks, a significant reduction (36.0% decrease) in the post–adrenocorticotropic hormone cortisol level.[32] However, Cortavance did not have any effect on peripheral CCR4$^+$CD4$^+$ T-lymphocytes.[32] Altogether, these studies showed a significant beneficial clinical effect of Cortavance in the treatment of mild canine AD as preventive or as management therapy. In addition, they show a large margin of safety of Cortavance in both short-term and long-term treatment of canine AD.

An alternative to topical GCs is CIs (tacrolimus and cyclosporine). Only 3 RDBPCTs[33-35] have been published on the use of tacrolimus for localized lesions of AD in dogs, 2 of which[33,34] investigated the use of the 0.1% and 1[35] the 0.3% formulation. In all 3 studies, the use of tacrolimus, although expensive, was very promising in treating localized atopic lesions with minimal side effects. In all studies, most dogs enrolled were able to achieve a treatment success (defined as $\geq$50% reduction in clinical signs from baseline) after 4 or 12 weeks of treatment. Mild irritation was noticed in a minority of cases after application and a lack of hematological and biochemical changes was reported. Detectable levels of tacrolimus were present in the blood at the end of the study; however, tacrolimus concentration was below toxicity limits. When 0.3% tacrolimus ointment was used,[35] a fourfold increase in tacrolimus concentrations was observed in the blood of dogs using 0.3% ointment. Due to equal efficacy and lower blood levels of tacrolimus, the 0.1% ointment is recommended as a safer choice. Cyclosporine, another calcineurin inhibitor, has been recently investigated as a topical treatment option for canine AD.[36] In a placebo-controlled clinical study, the investigators showed a significant clinical efficacy (localized lesions of moderate-severe AD) and moderate speed of action (21 days) of a nanotechnology pharmaceutical formulation of cyclosporine able to penetrate the epidermis, guaranteeing good absorption and dermal action. On days 21 and 45 after treatment, a significant reduction in clinical and pruritus score was seen in the treatment group compared with placebo, showing a rapid and effective action of the nano-compound in absence of side effects. However, more studies are needed to confirm the beneficial effect of this formulation in affected dogs.

Without a doubt, new-generation GCs and CIs are the most effective topical anti-inflammatory drugs used in canine AD. They are not only able to interfere with the in-flammatory cascade, but also decrease pruritus. However, due to cost or potential side effects, their use may be limited. Good alternative medications that can be used as glucocorticoid-sparing drugs include topical antihistamines, local anesthetics, and skin barrier–repairing agents.

Antihistamines (H1 receptor antagonists) acts on histamine receptors, competitively blocking the formation of histamine-receptor complex.[25] Thus, they inhibit the hista-minic cascade after histamine is released, with some antihistamines able to inhibit mast cell degranulation as well.[37] Common antihistamines used in veterinary derma-tology include diphenhydramine, hydroxyzine, and cetirizine. Although inexpensive and extremely safe, their efficacy has been historically low in treating allergic condi-tions in dogs; however, the lack of efficacy of antihistamine in canine AD may be because histamine is not the major player in cutaneous inflammation in atopic dogs and also because antihistamines are not able to dislodge histamine from its receptors once they are bound.[21,22,37] Unfortunately, the efficacy of topical H1 (diphenhydra-mine) and H4 (JNJ7777120 and JNJ28307474) antagonists has been shown to be low in recent studies.[38,39] Topical diphenhydramine was able to reduce clinical signs of AD only approximately 20% to 38% after 28 and 56 days of use, respectively.[38] Similarly, H4 antagonists, were not able to prevent skin lesions in a canine model of AD.[39] These 2 studies indicate a potential use of topical antihistamines in canine AD, although more studies are needed to fully evaluate the usefulness of such medi-ations in canine AD.

Local anesthetics have been used in clinical practice to alleviate the clinical signs of allergic dermatoses in dogs. In particular, the use of pramoxine as shampoo or cream rinse is of common use, although not many clinical trials have been published on its efficacy in dogs.[40] Only 1 crossover open clinical trial has evaluated the efficacy of 2 topical formulations of pramoxine cream rinse (Relief, Bayer, Shawnee, KS, USA; Derma-Soote, Vetoquinol, Fort Worth, Tx, USA) in atopic dogs for a total of 4 weeks. At the end of the study, pramoxine was judged effective (51%–75% reduction in pru-ritus) by 41% of the owners. The pos-treatment antipruritic effects lasted for 48 hours.

SKIN BARRIER–REPAIRING AGENTS

The use of anti-inflammatory/antipruritic topical mediations is essential in the treat-ment of allergic conditions in dogs. However, recent studies have shown that a skin barrier alteration, primary and/or secondary in nature, is present in both human and canine atopic skin. These results have led researchers and clinicians to look into ther-apies focused on ameliorating the skin barrier defect in allergic patients. In particular, topical fatty acids[41–43] and (pro)ceramides[44–50] have been largely used as adjuvant therapies for the treatment of canine AD. A few studies have been published on the effects of topical skin barrier–repairing agents showing a normalization of the epidermal lipid lamellae and skin lipids. However, the clinical effects of such products have been demonstrated in only a few clinical trials, showing an overall mild to mod-erate efficacy.

The use of essential fatty acids (EFAs), as adjuvant therapy for allergic skin condi-tions and dry skin, has been adapted in the clinical practice for decades. Essential fatty acids, in form of ω-3 and/or ω-6, have been administered as oral supplementation or through commercially available EFA-enriched diets. Only recently, the use of essential oil topical products has been considered as a potential alternative for delivering unsaturated EFA to affected skin. In 2011, an 8-week RDBPCT[41] was performed in Germany comparing the clinical effects of a spot-on formulation containing essential oils and unsaturated fatty acids (Dermoscent Essential 6 spot-on, Adventix, Burlington, ON, Canada) with a spray containing similar, although different, oils and fatty acids (Dermoscent Atop 7 spray). The outcomes measured included a clinical assessment, pruritus score, and skin barrier assessment (TEWL) at the beginning and at the end of the study. At the end of the study, there was a significant reduction in clinical signs (40% and 79% for spot-on and spray, respectively), pruritus score (32% and 43%), and TEWL (spray formulation). Finally, no side effects were reported for any of the treatments. The same research group performed another RDBPCT[42] analyzing the effects of the spot-on formulation against placebo over an 8-week period. The dogs were divided in mildly or moderately/severely affected atopic dogs. At the end of the study, a significant improvement of clinical signs and pruritus was seen in the treatment group. More recently, another RDBPCT43 evaluating the use of a topical lipid emulsion containing ceramides, fatty acids, and 18-β-glycyrrhetinic acid over a 3-month period was published. After the first month, a reduction of $\geq$50% in pruritus score was achieved in 50% of dogs; however, this beneficial effect was lost at the 3-month mark.

An alternative to essential oils and fatty acid topical formulations is the use of topical products containing a combination of ceramides, cholesterols, and fatty acids. In fact, early studies in people showed that products containing a specific molar ratio of ceramide, cholesterol, and fatty acids (3:1:1) to mimic the ratio naturally present in the skin were highly beneficial to improve skin lesions in atopic patients. In veterinary medicine, the first study[44] showing a beneficial effect of a spot-on product containing such molar ratio was published in 2008. In that study,[44] the investigators used a spot-on formulation (Allerderm spot-on by Virbac) every 3 days for 6 consecutive times. After 6 treatments, a significant reorganization of the intracorneal lipids, due to a possible increase in production and secretion of endogenous stratum corneum lipids, was seen. Another proof-of-concept study[49] was performed a few years later analyzing the expression of ceramides, cholesterol, and fatty acids in the stratum corneum of atopic dogs before and after 6 applications of Allerderm spot-on. At the end of the study, the investigators reported a significant increase in ceramide content and a more homogeneous distribution of protein-bound lipid content in the stratum corneum compared with before treatment. These studies were followed by 2 clinical trials evaluating the clinical benefits of Allerderm spot-on on atopic dogs[45,46]; both studies gave similar results. The use of Allerderm spot-on, applied twice weekly for 4 to 12 weeks, was associated with a significant decrease in clinical signs compared with baseline scores; however, no benefits were seen for pruritus and barrier function (TEWL). These studies demonstrated that the application of such products might improve the lipid biosynthesis and distribution in the stratum corneum ameliorating the skin barrier, however, its usefulness in clinical practice still needs additional studies.

The results obtained by Allerderm spot-on were confirmed by a more recent study[47] assessing the clinical and ultrastructural changes in atopic dogs before and after application of ceramide-based moisturizers for 28 days. The treatment involved the daily use of a moisturizing cream containing ceramide, cholesterol, and fatty acids (ration 3:1:1) (Atobarrier Cream, Aestura, Hangang-daero, Yongsan-gu, Seoul, Seoul, Korea) associated with a weekly moisturizing shampoo (Dermally shampoo, Dechra, Laewood, KS, USA). At the end of the study, a significant decrease in clinical signs, pruritus, and TEWL associated with an increase in skin hydration was reported. As far as the ultrastructural study, it showed a significant increase in thickness and continuity of the lipid bilayer.

Other skin barrier–repairing products that have increased in popularity in the past few years are topicals containing plant-derived sphingosines (phytosphingosines). Sphingosines are natural derivates of ceramides that have been associated with significant anti-inflammatory, antimicrobial, and barrier-repairing activity. A recent study in France[48] evaluated the barrier-repairing activity of a mousse containing phytosphingosines, raspberry oil, and lipids (Douxo Calm mousse, Ceva, Paris, France) in an experimental canine model. At the end of the study, there were no significant changes in TEWL or pH; however, a significant reduction of proliferation markers (ki-67) and B-lymphocytes and dendritic cells (BLA36) was seen in the treated compared with the untreated skin, suggesting a significant effect of phytosphingosines on inflammation and proliferation.

Altogether, these studies have shown that topical skin barrier–repairing agents have a significant benefit in treating canine AD. In particular, they are able to reduce cutaneous inflammation and restore intracorneal lipids normalizing the skin barrier of atopic dogs.

SYSTEMIC THERAPIES

Many systemic therapies have been investigated and routinely used in dogs affected by AD. As for the topical medications, it is important to recognize pros and cons of systemic therapies. The most important limitations of these drugs are cost, side effects, and lag phase. Because of their diversity in lag phases, some therapeutic options are more suitable for treating acute flares (eg, GC, oclacitinib), whereas others are more indicated for maintenance and/or prevention of flares (eg, allergen-specific immunotherapy, cyclosporine, antihistamines). This section is more focused on novel therapies (oclacitinib and lokivetmab) with a brief update on older therapies (cyclosporine).

Oclacitinib is a Janus kinase (JAK) inhibitor recently approved for treatment of allergic pruritus in dogs. There are 4 main types of JAK[51] present in mammalian cells (JAK1, JAK2, JAK3, and TYK2). Of those, JAK1 is the JAK mainly involved in the inflammatory response, whereas JAK2 and 3 and TYK2 are mainly involved in cell differentiation, hematopoiesis, and homeostasis.[51] Mechanistically, once a cytokine binds to the specific receptor, this dimerizes, allowing the autophosphorylation of JAK leading to the activation of the signal intermediate signal transducer and activator of transcription (STAT) proteins.[51] Once activated, STAT proteins (7 STATs have been identified in mammalian cells) will migrate to the nucleus, leading to DNA transcription and regulation of gene expression.[52,53] JAK/STAT signaling is critical for cytokine signaling and signal transduction of many proinflammatory, pro-allergic, and pruritogenic cytokines (eg, interleukin [IL]-2, IL-4, IL-6, IL-13, and IL-31).[54] Oclacitinib had increased popularity almost immediately after its lunch on the US market due to its rapid action associated with few side effects. Oclacitinib is mainly a JAK1 and 2 inhibitor; however, a slight affinity for TYR2 and JAK3 has been reported as well.[55] Its affinity profile explains the significant inhibition of inflammatory cytokines (IL-2, IL-4, IL-6, IL-13, and IL-31) and a minimal effect on hematopoietic cytokines (erythropoietin, granulocyte/macrophage colony-stimulating factor, IL-12, and IL-23).[55] Pharmacologically,[54] oclacitinib maleate is rapidly (plasmatic peak <1 hour) and almost completely (bioavailability of 89%) absorbed orally, independently from the prandial state, with a half-life of 4 to 6 hours, and a lack of cumulative effect over 168 days. Because of its speed of action, oclacitinib has been compared wwith prednisolone and dexamethasone in an experimental canine model of pruritus in which IL-31 was injected after the administration of each drug.[56] Prednisolone was able to inhibit the induced pruritus when administered 10 hours before the administration of IL-31, dexamethasone was able to reduce the pruritus up to 10 hours before IL-31 administration, whereas oclacitinib inhibited IL-31-induced pruritus when given 1, 6, 11, and 16 hours before IL-31 administration, making these compounds very similar from the clinical point of view. As far as efficacy, few studies[57–62] have assessed the clinical benefits and side effects of oclacitinib in treating allergic skin diseases in dogs. The first 2 studies[57,58] were very similar and showed that oclacitinib is a powerful drug, mainly active against pruritus. Oclacitinib was able to significantly reduce the pruritus within 7 days, with some improvement evident within 24 hours from administration.[57] In the second study, oclacitinib was administered for 112 days.[58] Over 28 days of treatment, a reduction in the pruritus score of 47.4% and 10.4% was detected in the oclacitinib and placebo groups, respectively; a reduction of 29.5% and 6.5% was seen within the first day of administration. From days 28 to 112, both the pruritus and clinical lesion scores remained unchanged. Minimal clinical and hematological abnormalities were reported in both studies. These studies were followed by a long-term compassionate use study[59] combining the information from dogs previously exposed to oclacitinib for a mean time of 401 days. The side effects reported in this study were also very similar to previous findings, highlighting the possibility of urinary tract infections, vomiting, otitis, pyoderma, and diarrhea. Four percent of dogs (mean age: 9.8 years) were euthanized because of confirmed or suspected malignancy. In addition, 19% of dogs developed new dermal, epidermal, or subcutaneous masses of unknown origin. There were no hematological abnormalities reported in the study.

Based on these exciting preliminary data, oclacitinib has significantly increased in popularity among clinicians, posing the question of whether oclacitinib would be more beneficial in treating AD than older systemic therapies such as GCs and cyclosporine. Thus, a first study[60] compared the use of oclacitinib with prednisolone over 28 days. Once again, pruritus and clinical signs were assessed, showing no difference between the 2 treatments after 4 hours, 6 days, and 18 days.[60] On the opposite hand, as expected, oclacitinib performed much better than cyclosporine in another prospective RDBPCT over 84 days of treatment at label doses.[61] In that study, a significantly higher reduction in pruritus score was seen in the oclacitinib group on days 1, 14, and 28, whereas a significant difference was seen only on day 14 for the clinical score. Because of the well-known long lag phase of cyclosporine, more recently, a study[62] evaluated the combined use of oclacitinib and cyclosporine, assessing the clinical safety of such combination over a 21-day trial. At the end of the study,[62] the investigators did not report any abnormalities except diarrhea in 2 dogs receiving both drugs.

Again, due to the numerous similarities between oclacitinib, GCs, and cyclosporine, potential complications (urinary tract infections),[63,64] reported in long-term use of these latter 2 medications, were evaluated for oclacitinib in a very recent study.[65] In that study, dogs receiving oclacitinib over 180 to 230 days did not show any signs (clinical or microbiological) of urinary tract infections. These studies indicate the usefulness of oclacitinib as good and safe alternative to other immunomodulatory drugs routinely used in veterinary dermatology to treat adult dogs affected by AD (eg, GC and cyclosporine).

Another treatment option that has acquired increasing popularity in treating canine AD is a caninized monoclonal anti-canine IL-31 antibody: lokivetmab. Lokivetmab was designed based on a recent study[66] showing a role of IL-31 in canine pruritus using a canine experimental model. However, whether IL-31 plays a significant role in canine AD is still controversial. In fact, in the original study,[66] only 57% of dogs with naturally occurring AD (detection limit 13 pg/mL) had a detectable serum level of IL-31. However, in a more recent study,[67] using a canine model of AD, the investigators were able to detect IL-31 in all the samples analyzed (~40–50 pg/mL) and similar results were recently presented[68] at the European Veterinary Dermatology Meeting showing the presence of IL-31 in the serum of 243 privately owned atopic dogs and 55 normal dogs using a more advanced ultrasensitive enzyme-linked immunosorbent assay technology able to detect extremely low amounts of protein in serum (femtomolar level of 531 fg/mL and 13,541 fg/mL in healthy and atopic dogs, respectively).

Lokivetmab is the first biologic commercially available for the treatment of allergic conditions in dogs. Its mechanism of action is quite simple: once injected, lokivetmab recognizes and binds to naturally produced IL-31, making it unavailable to bind to its receptor and trigger the pruritic cascade. Because foreign antibodies are readily recognized by the host's immune system and destroyed, lokivetmab was made fully caninized (90% or more of the antibody structure is similar to antibody produced naturally in dogs) so as to avoid recognition and last longer. This type of technology has been largely used in human medicine to make humanized monoclonal antibodies to treat several immunologically driven diseases (eg, rheumatoid arthritis, psoriasis, AD). Since lokivetmab was initially commercialized, a few clinical studies[69–71] have been published assessing its efficacy and safety in atopic dogs.

The first study involved atopic dogs throughout the United States.[69] Dogs were assigned to receive a single subcutaneous injection of different dose of lokivetmab (0.125, 03.5, and 2 mg/kg) or placebo and monitored for clinical efficacy (pruritus and clinical signs) for 56 days. At full dose, a significant decrease in pruritus score was seen within 1 to 3 days, followed by a decrease in clinical signs after only 7 days. After 28 days, the success rate for the pruritus (decrease of ≥50% in score compared with baseline) was between 21% and 57%, depending on the dose used. Similarly, the success rate for the clinical score varied between 13% and 46% based on the dosage. Furthermore, pharmacokinetic data showed that, at full dose, the mean peak serum concentration of lokivetmab is 10 µg/mL observed after 9.8 days (2 mg/kg) with a mean half-life of 16 days.[69] Similar results were evident from a clinical field trial[70,71] evaluating the long-term efficacy and safety of lokivetmab for atopic dogs. In that study, lokivetmab was administered to atopic dogs for 9 consecutive months at monthly intervals. At the end of the trial, 76% of dogs were assessed as being "normal,"whereas 59% were assessed as clinically "in remission." Mild side effects were recorded and no immunogenicity (ie, anti-lokivetmab antibody development) was seen in any dog. Finally, a noninferiority study[71] compared the efficacy of lokivetmab with cyclosporine. In that study, atopic dogs were enrolled and assigned to receive monthly lokivetmab or daily oral cyclosporine for 3 months. Lokivetmab was not inferior to cyclosporine for either pruritus or clinical signs, with an overall response to treatment of 68.5% and 72.5% by the owner and 74.0% and 72.9% by the investigator for cyclosporine and lokivetmab, respectively.

These studies altogether show that lokivetmab is a safe and effective treatment alternative to systemic GC and cyclosporine.

Cyclosporine has been considered a good GC-sparing agent for the past 20 years. Many of the clinical studies, proving the efficacy and safety of cyclosporine in dogs affected by AD, have been published in the past 2 decades. Cyclosporine is widely recognized to be highly effective in the treatment of canine AD and associated with minimal side effects. The author refers the reader to previously published reviews on cyclosporine efficacy in atopic dogs.[72–77]

Recent studies have been mainly focused on the effects of cyclosporine on skin barrier function, skin microbiota, and effect on T-cell subtypes. In particular, one open study[78] analyzed the effects of cyclosporine on TEWL, as indirect measurement of skin barrier integrity, in severely affected atopic dogs. The investigators were able to show that although a significant decrease in clinical signs was present after the second week on treatment, a significant decrease in TEWL, in selected areas, was detected from the first week on cyclosporine. Another single-blinded, randomized, placebo-controlled study[79] evaluated the effect of cyclosporine on skin barrier integrity on a colony of atopic beagles before and after chronic stimulation with house dust mites. In that study, the investigators showed that 28 days of cyclosporine did not have any significant effect on skin immunologic milieu (IL-2, IL-4, IL-10, IL-13, interferon-γ, tumor necrosis factor-α, and transforming growth factor-β) or skin barrier markers (canine antimicrobial peptides, filaggrin 2, and caspase 14) despite evident improvement of physical signs. Similarly, a lack of effect of cyclosporine on the skin microbiota was evident from another recent study[80] using Maltese-beagle atopic dogs. In particular, the investigators showed that both cyclosporine and prednisone administered for 1 month were not associated with any significant changes in the cutaneous microbiota (bacteria, fungi, and viruses). Finally, very recently, the effect of cyclosporine on lymphocyte subpopulations also has been investigated to better understand the specific immunomodulatory effect of this compound on the immune system. In that controlled study,[81] the investigators showed that 90 days of cyclosporine therapy, although significantly decreasing the clinical signs, did not modify the circulating T-cell ratio (CD4/CD8) and number of T-regulatory cells in atopic dogs. Thus, new studies have confirmed the beneficial clinical effect of cyclosporine for atopic dogs, but also showed that this compound has little effect on alteration of skin barrier, lymphocytic subpopulations, and cutaneous microbiota in atopic dogs.

ALTERNATIVE THERAPIES

The research of alternative therapies to treat canine AD has seen a tremendous increase in the past decade. In particular, researchers have invested in searching for more natural compounds with fewer side effects able to reduce or completely eliminate the needs of medications generally used for AD (eg, GC, cyclosporine, oclacitinib). The earliest and most repeated attempt was done looking into probiotics as a potential tool to reduce or prevent clinical signs of AD in dogs.[82–86] In particular, the use of *Lactobacillus rhamnosus* has been shown to be effective in preventing the development of AD in a canine model when given in utero (from the third week of gestation until lactation) and continued in the offspring from the third week to 6 months of age.[82] Immunologic and structural (skin barrier function) benefits were still evident after 3 years from the administration.[83,84] More recently, a study,[85] comparing cetirizine with *Lactobacillus paracasei K71*, showed a similar reduction in clinical signs (38.1% vs 45.8%) and pruritus (38.1% vs 26.8%) scores in mild cases of AD over 12 weeks of treatment. Similar results were confirmed by using *Lactobacillus sakei probio-65* after 8 weeks in dogs with severe AD.[86] Altogether, these studies suggest that the administration of probiotics could be beneficial in preventing or reducing the clinical signs (and drugs) of AD in dogs. However, it is essential to keep in mind that not all bacteria act as probiotics, and particular attention needs to be applied to the choice of probiotics to be administered to optimize their beneficial effects.

Other treatments reported to be useful in reducing the clinical signs or the need of drugs to treat atopic dogs have been studied. In particular, oral vitamin E, associated with fexofenadine, has been shown to be highly effective in reducing clinical signs in moderate cases of AD after 8 weeks of treatment when compared with placebo plus fexofenadine (96% vs 89%, respectively).[87] The investigators also reported an increase in circulating vitamin E and an increase in total antioxidant capacity. Similarly, the use of oral vitamin D has been shown to be promising when used in mild to moderate cases of AD for 8 weeks.[88] As in the vitamin E study, an increase in circulating vitamin D was detected. In both studies, a lack of side effects was reported.

Other alternative therapies shown to be effective in the treatment of canine AD include the use of procaine (neural therapy), ultrapure water, pentoxifylline plus polyunsaturated fatty acids (PUFAs), and endocannabinoids, whereas other options have not been associated with a significant or questionable improvement of canine AD (eg, cold laser therapy, homeopathy, fluoxetine, CCR4 inhibitors, aminopterin) or associated with moderate to severe side effects (eg, masitinib).

Briefly, the use of procaine intravenously and intradermally (in affected areas), showed a significant reduction of 82.6% and 77.4% in clinical signs and pruritus score with 88% of dogs reaching a reduction of both scores of $\geq$50% after 13 weeks of treatment in absence of side effects.[89] Furthermore, a maintained improvement of the clinical signs was seen in 55% of the dogs enrolled after 19 weeks from last injection.

Recently, a placebo-controlled clinical trial[90] evaluated the efficacy of weekly Allermyl shampoo (ceramides and EFAs) using ultrapure soft water compared with Allermyl shampoo using tap water in moderate cases of canine AD over a 4-week period. Ultrapure soft water is characterized by low hardness, low calcium and magnesium, and high sodium compared with tap water. The study showed a significant decrease in clinical signs (21% vs −0.45%), pruritus (24.0% vs 3.6%), and TEWL (46.4% vs −6.0%) for the treatment group compared with the control.

Pentoxifylline is a nonselective phosphodiesterase enzyme inhibitor able to decrease fibronectin, production of proinflammatory cytokines, and leukocyte response to interleukins, and impairs T-lymphocyte binding to keratinocytes, decreases fibroblastic activity, and with long-term use, may decrease fibrosis. Although clinically used, only 1 placebo-controlled, randomized study[91] has been published assessing its efficacy in treating canine AD. Pentoxifylline was administered orally at the dosage of 20 mg/kg every 8 hours, alone (group I) or in combination with oral PUFAs (group II), for 60 days. On days 30 and 60, a significant reduction in both clinical signs and pruritus scores was seen in both treatment groups compared with placebo (group III) and with baseline. However, the combination of pentoxifylline and PUFAs was more efficacious than pentoxifylline alone.

Last, the oral use of naturally occurring bioactive lipid endocannabinoidlike compounds has been investigated in dogs affected by AD. In particular, an open-label clinical trial[92] using ultra-micronized palmitoylethanolamide at 10.9 mg/kg per day for 8 weeks showed a significant reduction in both clinical signs (day 28: 31.6%; day 56: 48.2%) and pruritus (day 28: 26%; day 56: 36.8%), and an increase in quality of life. This study, although it is the first one published in dogs, is very promising.

As far as homeopathic remedies for treating AD in dogs, only 1 small pilot study showed a potential benefit of individualized remedies in canine AD.[93] However, due to the very low number of dogs enrolled and the lack of a controlled, blinded, randomized clinical trial, the use of homeopathy is not justified at the moment. The use of cold laser therapy was investigated in a placebo-controlled, clinical trial.[94] However, after 5 weeks of treatment, no difference in clinical signs and pruritus was present between low-level laser therapy (cold laser) and placebo. Finally, a double-blinded, placebo-controlled crossover 2-month clinical trial[95] evaluated the efficacy of fluoxetine for severe AD, showing no efficacy after 2 months of fluoxetine.

FUTURE THERAPIES

Looking at the future, it is possible that safer and more targeted compounds will be available for canine AD. Specifically, biologics targeting molecules involved in the treatment of specific clinical subtypes of AD are desirable.[96] On the other hand, the use of viral-particle-associated cytokines[97] or bacterins[98,99] have also been studied as potential treatments for allergies in animals. Their efficacy is variable but promising in the face of mild side effects. Among others, humanized anti-interleukin antibodies (targeting IL-4, IL-13, IL-17, and IL-22) have been studied, or are currently under evaluation, for the treatment of human AD. Along with anti-interleukin antibodies, the use of anti-human IgE and anti–IL-31 receptor antibodies have been highly promising as well. In veterinary medicine, the only biologic approved is lokivetmab. It is plausible to assume that more biologics will be readily available in the near future; however, based on the complexity of the atopic disease, instead of a single monoclonal antibody, maybe the use of cocktails of monoclonal antibodies may increase the efficacy of this therapeutic option.

SUMMARY

In conclusion, canine AD is an extremely complex clinical syndrome characterized by different clinical manifestations and therapeutic response. Because of its complexity, multiple therapies have been evaluated in different clinical subtypes, with sometimes contrasting results. At the moment, a pool of few compounds represent the "core" of treatment options for canine AD (eg, GC, cyclosporine, oclacitinib). However, alternative drugs and topical therapies have been looked at with increased interest due to their low toxicity and high efficacy, specifically if associated with "core" medications. Furthermore, it is fundamental to remember to strive for preventive medicine using compounds able to delay rather that treat flares and skin infections in atopic dogs. In addition, it is important to recognize the difference in drugs more suited for treating flares and drugs more effective in preventing the flares. Treatment options should be regularly reassessed and adjusted based on the specific needs of patients and their owners. The key of a successful treatment for canine AD often combines high efficacy with low cost and mild side effects.

REFERENCES

1. Halliwell R. Revised nomenclature for veterinary allergy. Vet Immunol Immunopathol 2006;114:207–8.
2. Prelaud P, Cochet-Faivre N. A retrospective study of 21 cases of canine atopic-like dermatitis. Vet Dermatol 2007;18:385.
3. Botoni LS, Torres SMF, Kock SN, et al. Comparison of clinical and epidemiological features of canine atopic dermatitis and atopic-like dermatitis: a retrospective study. Vet Dermatol 2018;29:8.
4. Fujimura M, Nakatsuji Y, Ishimaru H. Cyclosporin A treatment in intrinsic canine atopic dermatitis (atopic-like dermatitis): open trial study. Pol J Vet Sci 2016;19:567–72.
5. Marsella R, De Benedetto A. Atopic dermatitis in animals and people: an update and comparative review. Vet Sci 2017;4 [pii:E37].
6. Hillier A, Griffin CE. The ACVD task force on canine atopic dermatitis (I): incidence and prevalence. Vet Immunol Immunopathol 2001;81:147–51.
7. Hill PB, Lo A, Eden CA, et al. Survey of the prevalence, diagnosis and treatment of dermatological conditions in small animals in general practice. Vet Rec 2006;158:533–9.
8. Nodtvedt A, Egenvall A, Bergvall K, et al. Incidence of and risk factors for atopic dermatitis in a Swedish population of insured dogs. Vet Rec 2006;159:241–6.

9. Jaeger K, Linek M, Power HT, et al. Breed and site predispositions of dogs with atopic dermatitis: a comparison of five locations in three continents. Vet Dermatol 2009;21:119–23.

10. Santoro D, Marsella R, Hernandez J. Investigation on the association between atopic dermatitis and the development of mycosis fungoides in dogs: a retrospective case-control study. Vet Dermatol 2007;18:101–6.

11. Sousa CA, Marsella R. The ACVD task force on canine atopic dermatitis (II): genetic factors. Vet Immunol Immunopathol 2001;81:153–7.

12. Hensel P, Santoro D, Favrot C, et al. Canine atopic dermatitis: detailed guidelines for diagnosis and allergen identification. BMC Vet Res 2015;11:196.

13. Wilhem S, Kovalik M, Favrot C. Breed-associated phenotypes in canine atopic dermatitis. Vet Dermatol 2011;22:143–9.

14. Pucheu-Haston CM, Eisenschenk MN, Bizikova P, et al. Introduction to the review articles by ICADA on the pathogenesis of atopic dermatitis in dogs. Vet Dermatol 2015;26:77–8.

15. Bizikova P, Santoro D, Marsella R, et al. Review: clinical and histological manifestations of canine atopic dermatitis. Vet Dermatol 2015;26:79-e24.

16. Santoro D, Marsella R, Pucheu-Haston CM, et al. Review: pathogenesis of canine atopic dermatitis: skin barrier and host-micro-organism interaction. Vet Dermatol 2015;26:84-e25.

17. Bizikova P, Pucheu-Haston CM, Eisenschenk MN, et al. Review: role of genetics and the environment in the pathogenesis of canine atopic dermatitis. Vet Dermatol 2015;26:95-e26.

18. Pucheu-Haston CM, Santoro D, Bizikova P, et al. Review: innate immunity, lipid metabolism and nutrition in canine atopic dermatitis. Vet Dermatol 2015;26:104-e28.

19. Pucheu-Haston CM, Bizikova P, Eisenschenk MN, et al. Review: the role of antibodies, autoantigens and food allergens in canine atopic dermatitis. Vet Dermatol 2015;26:115-e30.

20. Pucheu-Haston CM, Bizikova P, Marsella R, et al. Review: lymphocytes, cytokines, chemokines and the T-helper 1-T-helper 2 balance in canine atopic dermatitis. Vet Dermatol 2015;26:124-e32.

21. Olivry T, DeBoer DJ, Favrot C, et al. Treatment of canine atopic dermatitis: 2010 clinical practice guidelines from the International Task Force on Canine Atopic Dermatitis. Vet Dermatol 2010;21:233–48.

22. Olivry T, DeBoer DJ, Favrot C, et al. Treatment of canine atopic dermatitis: 2015 updated guidelines from the International Committee on Allergic Diseases of Animals (ICADA). BMC Vet Res 2015;11:210.

23. Loeflath A, von Voigts-Rhetz A, Jaeger K, et al. The use of a whirlpool in topical antipruritic therapy–a double-blinded, randomized, cross-over study. Vet Dermatol 2007;18:427–31.

24. Reme CA, Mondon A, Calmon JP, et al. Efficacy of combined topical therapy with antiallergic shampoo and lotion for the control of signs associated with atopic dermatitis in dogs. Vet Dermatol 2004;15:S33.

25. Olivry T, Bäumer W. Atopic itch in dogs: pharmacology and modeling. Handb Exp Pharmacol 2015;226:357–69.

26. Deboer DJ, Schafer JH, Salsbury CS, et al. Multiple-center study of reduced-concentration triamcinolone topical solution for the treatment of dogs with known or suspected allergic pruritus. Am J Vet Res 2002;63:408–13.

27. Nuttall T, Mueller R, Bensignor E, et al. Efficacy of a 0.0584% hydrocortisone aceponate spray in the management of canine atopic dermatitis: a randomised, double blind, placebo-controlled trial. Vet Dermatol 2009;20:191–8.
28. Nuttall TJ, McEwan NA, Bensignor E, et al. Comparable efficacy of a topical 0.0584% hydrocortisone aceponate spray and oral ciclosporin in treating canine atopic dermatitis. Vet Dermatol 2012;23:4–10, e1–2.
29. Nam EH, Park SH, Jung JY, et al. Evaluation of the effect of a 0.0584% hydrocortisone aceponate spray on clinical signs and skin barrier function in dogs with atopic dermatitis. J Vet Sci 2012;13:187–91.
30. Lourenço AM, Schmidt V, São Braz B, et al. Efficacy of proactive long-term maintenance therapy of canine atopic dermatitis with 0.0584% hydrocortisone aceponate spray: a double-blind placebo controlled pilot study. Vet Dermatol 2016;27: 88–92e25.
31. Bizikova P, Linder KE, Paps J, et al. Effect of a novel topical diester glucocorticoid spray on immediate- and late-phase cutaneous allergic reactions in Maltese-beagle atopic dogs: a placebo-controlled study. Vet Dermatol 2010; 21:70–9.
32. Fujimura M, Ishimaru H. Influence of a diester glucocorticoid spray on the cortisol level and the CCR4(+) CD4(+) lymphocytes in dogs with atopic dermatitis: open study. J Vet Med 2014;2014:492735.
33. Marsella R, Nicklin CF, Saglio S, et al. Investigation on the clinical efficacy and safety of 0.1% tacrolimus ointment (Protopic) in canine atopic dermatitis: a randomized, double-blinded, placebo-controlled, cross-over study. Vet Dermatol 2004;15:294–303.
34. Bensignor E, Olivry T. Treatment of localized lesions of canine atopic dermatitis with tacrolimus ointment: a blinded randomized controlled trial. Vet Dermatol 2005;16:52–60.
35. Marsella R, Nicklin CF. Investigation on the use of 0.3% tacrolimus lotion for canine atopic dermatitis: a pilot study. Vet Dermatol 2002;13:203–10.
36. Puigdemont A, Brazís P, Ordeix L, et al. Efficacy of a new topical cyclosporine A formulation in the treatment of atopic dermatitis in dogs. Vet J 2013;197:280–5.
37. DeBoer DJ, Griffin CE. The ACVD task force on canine atopic dermatitis (XXI): antihistamine pharmacotherapy. Vet Immunol Immunopathol 2001;81:323–9.
38. Iwasaki T, Hasegawa A. A randomized comparative clinical trial of recombinant canine interferon-gamma (KT-100) in atopic dogs using antihistamine as control. Vet Dermatol 2006;17:195–200.
39. Bäumer W, Stahl J, Sander K, et al. Lack of preventing effect of systemically and topically administered histamine H(1) or H(4) receptor antagonists in a dog model of acute atopic dermatitis. Exp Dermatol 2011;20:577–81.
40. Scott DW, Rothstein E, Miller WH. A clinical study on the efficacy of two commercial veterinary pramoxine cream rinses in the management of pruritus in atopic dogs. Canine Pract 2000;25:15–7.
41. Tretter S, Mueller RS. The influence of topical unsaturated fatty acids and essential oils on normal and atopic dogs. J Am Anim Hosp Assoc 2011;47:236–40.
42. Blaskovic M, Rosenkrantz W, Neuber A, et al. The effect of a spot-on formulation containing polyunsaturated fatty acids and essential oils on dogs with atopic dermatitis. Vet J 2014;199:39–43.
43. Marsella R, Cornegliani L, Ozmen I, et al. Randomized, double-blinded, placebo-controlled pilot study on the effects of topical black currant emulsion enriched in essential fatty acids, ceramides and 18-beta glycyrrhetinic acid on clinical signs

and skin barrier function in dogs with atopic dermatitis. Vet Dermatol 2017;28: 577-e140.

44. Piekutowska A, Pin D, Rème CA, et al. Effects of a topically applied preparation of epidermal lipids on the stratum corneum barrier of atopic dogs. J Comp Pathol 2008;138:197–203.

45. Fujimura M, Nakatsuji Y, Fujiwara S, et al. Spot-on skin lipid complex as an adjuvant therapy in dogs with atopic dermatitis: an open pilot study. Vet Med Int 2011; 2011:281846.

46. Marsella R, Genovese D, Gilmer L, et al. Investigations on the effects of a topical ceramides-containing emulsion (Allerderm® Spot on) on clinical signs and skin barrier function in dogs with atopic dermatitis: a double-blinded, randomized, controlled study. Intern J Appl Res Vet Med 2013;2:110–6.

47. Jung JY, Nam EH, Park SH, et al. Clinical use of a ceramide-based moisturizer for treating dogs with atopic dermatitis. J Vet Sci 2013;14:199–205.

48. Pin D, Bekrich M, Fantini O, et al. An emulsion restores the skin barrier by decreasing the skin pH and inflammation in a canine experimental model. J Comp Pathol 2014;151:244–54.

49. Popa I, Remoue N, Osta B, et al. The lipid alterations in the stratum corneum of dogs with atopic dermatitis are alleviated by topical application of a sphingolipid-containing emulsion. Clin Exp Dermatol 2012;37:665–71.

50. Cerrato S, Ramió-Lluch L, Brazís P, et al. Effects of sphingolipid extracts on the morphological structure and lipid profile in an in vitro model of canine skin. Vet J 2016;212:58–64.

51. Cinats A, Heck E, Robertson L. Janus kinase inhibitors: a review of their emerging applications in dermatology. Skin Therapy Lett 2018;23:5–9.

52. O'Shea JJ, Holland SM, Staudt LM. JAKs and STATs in immunity, immunodeficiency, and cancer. N Engl J Med 2013;368:161–70.

53. Villarino AV, Kanno Y, Ferdinand JR, et al. Mechanisms of JAK/STAT signaling in immunity and disease. J Immunol 2015;194:21–7.

54. Collard WT, Hummel BD, Fielder AF, et al. The pharmacokinetics of oclacitinib maleate, a Janus Kinase inhibitor, in the dog. J Vet Pharmacol Ther 2014;37: 279–85.

55. Gonzales AJ, Bowman JW, Fici GJ, et al. Oclacitinib (APOQUEL®) is a novel Janus Kinase inhibitor with activity against cytokines involved in allergy. J Vet Pharmacol Ther 2014;37:317–24.

56. Gonzales AJ, Fleck TJ, Humphrey WR, et al. IL-31-induced pruritus in dogs: a novel experimental model to evaluate anti-pruritic effects of canine therapeutics. Vet Dermatol 2016;27:34-e10.

57. Cosgrove SB, Wren JA, Cleaver DM, et al. Efficacy and safety of oclacitinib for the control of pruritus and associated skin lesions in dogs with canine allergic dermatitis. Vet Dermatol 2013;24:479-e114.

58. Cosgrove SB, Wren JA, Cleaver DM, et al. A blinded, randomized, placebo-controlled trial of the efficacy and safety of the Janus kinase inhibitor oclacitinib (Apoquel®) in client-owned dogs with atopic dermatitis. Vet Dermatol 2013;24: 587-e142.

59. Cosgrove SB, Cleaver DM, King VL, et al. Long-term compassionate use of oclacitinib in dogs with atopic and allergic skin disease: safety, efficacy and quality of life. Vet Dermatol 2015;26:171-e35.

60. Gadeyne C, Little P, King VL, et al. Efficacy of oclacitinib (Apoquel®) compared with prednisolone for the control of pruritus and clinical signs associated with

    allergic dermatitis in client-owned dogs in Australia. Vet Dermatol 2014;25: 512-e86.

61. Little PR, King VL, Davis KR, et al. A blinded, randomized clinical trial comparing the efficacy and safety of oclacitinib and ciclosporin for the control of atopic dermatitis in client-owned dogs. Vet Dermatol 2015;26:23-e8.

62. Panteri A, Strehlau G, Helbig R, et al. Repeated oral dose tolerance in dogs treated concomitantly with ciclosporin and oclacitinib for three weeks. Vet Dermatol 2016;27:22-e7.

63. Peterson AL, Torres SM, Rendahl A, et al. Frequency of urinary tract infection in dogs with inflammatory skin disorders treated with ciclosporin alone or in combination with glucocorticoid therapy: a retrospective study. Vet Dermatol 2012;23: 201-e43.

64. Torres SM, Diaz SF, Nogueira SA, et al. Frequency of urinary tract infection among dogs with pruritic disorders receiving long-term glucocorticoid treatment. J Am Vet Med Assoc 2005;227:239–43.

65. Simpson AC, Schissler JR, Rosychuk RAW, et al. The frequency of urinary tract infection and subclinical bacteriuria in dogs with allergic dermatitis treated with oclacitinib: a prospective study. Vet Dermatol 2017;28:485-e113.

66. Gonzales AJ, Humphrey WR, Messamore JE, et al. Interleukin-31: its role in canine pruritus and naturally occurring canine atopic dermatitis. Vet Dermatol 2013;24:48-e12.

67. Marsella R, Ahrens K, Sanford R. Investigation of the correlation of serum IL-31 with severity of dermatitis in an experimental model of canine atopic dermatitis using beagle dogs. Vet Dermatol 2018;29:69-e28.

68. Messamore JE. An ultrasensitive single molecule array (Simoa) for the detection of IL-31 in canine serum shows differential levels in dogs affected with atopic dermatitis compared to healthy animals. Vet Dermatol 2017;28:546.

69. Michels GM, Ramsey DS, Walsh KF, et al. A blinded, randomized, placebo-controlled, dose determination trial of lokivetmab (ZTS-00103289), a caninized, anti-canine IL-31 monoclonal antibody in client owned dogs with atopic dermatitis. Vet Dermatol 2016;27:478-e129.

70. Moyaert H, Van Brussel L, Borowski S, et al. A clinical field trial evaluating the long-term efficacy and safety of lokivetmab in client owned dogs with atopic dermatitis. Vet Dermatol 2017;28:547.

71. Moyaert H, Van Brussel L, Borowski S, et al. A blinded, randomized clinical trial evaluating the efficacy and safety of lokivetmab compared to ciclosporin in client-owned dogs with atopic dermatitis. Vet Dermatol 2017;28:593-e145.

72. Nuttall T, Reece D, Roberts E. Life-long diseases need life-long treatment: long-term safety of ciclosporin in canine atopic dermatitis. Vet Rec 2014;174(S2): 3–12.

73. Forsythe P, Paterson S. Ciclosporin 10 years on: indications and efficacy. Vet Rec 2014;174(S2):13–21.

74. Archer TM, Boothe DM, Langston VC, et al. Oral cyclosporine treatment in dogs: a review of the literature. J Vet Intern Med 2014;28:1–20.

75. DeBoer DJ. Ciclosporin in canine dermatology: a decade of comfort. Vet Rec 2014;174(S2):1–2.

76. Palmeiro BS. Cyclosporine in veterinary dermatology. Vet Clin North Am Small Anim Pract 2013;43:153–71.

77. Kovalik M, Thoday KL, van den Broek AH. The use of ciclosporin A in veterinary dermatology. Vet J 2012;193:317–25.

78. Zając M, Szczepanik M, Wilkołek P, et al. The influence of non-specific anti-pruritus treatment with cyclosporine A on transepidermal water loss (TEWL) in natural atopic dermatitis in dogs. Pol J Vet Sci 2015;18:415–24.
79. White AG, Santoro D, Ahrens K, et al. Single blinded, randomized, placebo-controlled study on the effects of ciclosporin on cutaneous barrier function and immunological response in atopic beagles. Vet Immunol Immunopathol 2018; 197:93–101.
80. Widmer G, Ferrer L, Favrot C, et al. Glucocorticoids and cyclosporin do not significantly impact canine cutaneous microbiota. BMC Vet Res 2018;14:51.
81. Beccati M, Martini V, Comazzi S, et al. Lymphocyte subpopulations and Treg cells in dogs with atopic dermatitis receiving ciclosporin therapy: a prospective study. Vet Dermatol 2016;27:17-e5.
82. Marsella R. Evaluation of *Lactobacillus rhamnosus* strain GG for the prevention of atopic dermatitis in dogs. Am J Vet Res 2009;70:735–40.
83. Marsella R, Santoro D, Ahrens K. Early exposure to probiotics in a canine model of atopic dermatitis has long-term clinical and immunological effects. Vet Immunol Immunopathol 2012;146:185–9.
84. Marsella R, Santoro D, Ahrens K, et al. Investigation of the effect of probiotic exposure on filaggrin expression in an experimental model of canine atopic dermatitis. Vet Dermatol 2013;24:260-e57.
85. Ohshima-Terada Y, Higuchi Y, Kumagai T, et al. Complementary effect of oral administration of *Lactobacillus paracasei* K71 on canine atopic dermatitis. Vet Dermatol 2015;26:350-e75.
86. Kim H, Rather IA, Kim H, et al. A double-blind, placebo controlled-trial of a probiotic strain *Lactobacillus sakei* Probio-65 for the prevention of canine atopic dermatitis. J Microbiol Biotechnol 2015;25:1966–9.
87. Plevnik Kapun A, Salobir J, Levart A, et al. Vitamin E supplementation in canine atopic dermatitis: improvement of clinical signs and effects on oxidative stress markers. Vet Rec 2014;175:560.
88. Klinger CJ, Hobi S, Johansen C, et al. Vitamin D shows in vivo efficacy in a placebo-controlled, double-blinded, randomized clinical trial on canine atopic dermatitis. Vet Rec 2018;182:406.
89. Bravo-Monsalvo A, Vázquez-Chagoyán JC, Gutiérrez L, et al. Clinical efficacy of neural therapy for the treatment of atopic dermatitis in dogs. Acta Vet Hung 2008; 56:459–69.
90. Ohmori K, Tanaka A, Makita Y, et al. Pilot evaluation of the efficacy of shampoo treatment with ultrapure soft water for canine pruritus. Vet Dermatol 2010;21: 477–83.
91. Singh SK, Dimri U, Saxena SK, et al. Therapeutic management of canine atopic dermatitis by combination of pentoxifylline and PUFAs. J Vet Pharmacol Ther 2010;33:495–8.
92. Noli C, Della Valle MF, Miolo A, et al. Efficacy of ultra-micronized palmitoylethanolamide in canine atopic dermatitis: an open-label multi-centre study. Vet Dermatol 2015;26:432–40, e101.
93. Hill PB, Hoare J, Lau-Gillard P, et al. Pilot study of the effect of individualised homeopathy on the pruritus associated with atopic dermatitis in dogs. Vet Rec 2009;164:364–70.
94. Stich AN, Rosenkrantz WS, Griffin CE. Clinical efficacy of low-level laser therapy on localized canine atopic dermatitis severity score and localized pruritic visual analog score in pedal pruritus due to canine atopic dermatitis. Vet Dermatol 2014;25:464-e74.

95. Fujimura M, Ishimaru H, Nakatsuji Y. Fluoxetine (SSRI) treatment of canine atopic dermatitis: a randomized, double-blind, placebo-controlled, crossover trial. Pol J Vet Sci 2014;17:371–3.

96. Fabbrocini G, Napolitano M, Megna M, et al. Treatment of atopic dermatitis with biologic drugs. Dermatol Ther (Heidelb) 2018. [Epub ahead of print].

97. Fettelschoss-Gabriel A, Fettelschoss V, Thoms F, et al. Treating insect-bite hypersensitivity in horses with active vaccination against IL-5. J Allergy Clin Immunol 2018. [Epub ahead of print].

98. Ricklin Gutzwiller ME, Reist M, Peel JE, et al. Intradermal injection of heat-killed Mycobacterium vaccae in dogs with atopic dermatitis: a multicentre pilot study. Vet Dermatol 2007;18:87–93.

99. Marro A, Pirles M, Schiaffino L, et al. Successful immunotherapy of canine flea allergy with injected Actinomycetales preparations. Immunotherapy 2011;3: 971–8.

Sterile Pyogranulomatous Dermatitis and Panniculitis

Jennifer Schissler, DVM, MS

KEYWORDS

- Pyogranulomatous • Dermatitis • Ulcerative • Nodular • Sterile • Panniculitis

KEY POINTS

- The diagnosis involves exclusion of infectious causes of pyogranulomatous dermatitis and panniculitis via histopathology, tissue culture, and ancillary diagnostics.
- Prodromal and concurrent nonspecific clinical and hematologic signs of inflammation may occur.
- This syndrome is characterized by pyogranulomatous nodules, plaques, and ulcers of variable extent and severity.
- This syndrome is idiopathic and typically responds well to corticosteroids and corticosteroid-sparing immunomodulatory drugs.

INTRODUCTION

Canine nodular and ulcerative dermatitis is a diagnostic challenge. Bacterial infection, fungal infection, oomycosis, foreign bodies, and sterile inflammatory conditions may present similarly as solitary or multifocal cutaneous nodules, plaques, ulcers, and draining tracts with pyogranulomatous inflammation. A thorough physical examination and history aid in prioritization of differentials. The cause of the nodules and ulcers may be efficiently identified via cytology or may remain elusive, requiring histopathology, culture, and ancillary diagnostics.

Sterile pyogranulomatous dermatitis and panniculitis (SPDP) is an uncommon syndrome of adult and, rarely, juvenile dogs. No autoantigen, or exogenous antigen stimulus has been identified. SPDP is characterized by pyogranulomatous nodules, plaques, and ulcers of variable size, extent, and severity. This syndrome does not have a formalized name. Other terms used to describe this syndrome include: *sterile granuloma/pyogranuloma syndrome, sterile panniculitis, sterile granulomatous/pyogranulomatous dermatitis and panniculitis*. As indicated by the variation in

Disclosure Statement: The author has received remuneration from Zoetis for content delivered at continuing education events. The author has conducted research published in *Veterinary Dermatology* sponsored by Zoetis.
Department of Clinical Sciences, James L. Voss Veterinary Teaching Hospital, 300 West Drake Road, Fort Collins, CO 80525, USA
E-mail address: Jennifer.schissler@colostate.edu

vetsmall.theclinics.com

nomenclature, patients may demonstrate gross and histopathologic manifestations of dermatitis, panniculitis, or both.

SPDP is a diagnosis of exclusion. Treatment of SPDP requires systemic immuno-modulation. Therefore, misdiagnosis of SPDP and subsequent immunosuppressive treatment is ineffective, at best. At worst, misdiagnosis is catastrophically counterproductive. To successfully navigate pyogranulomatous and ulcerative dermatitis, a thorough and rational diagnostic approach is paramount.

SIGNALMENT AND HISTORY

Patients may present with an acute history involving singular or multiple cutaneous lesions as well as cutaneous pain, malaise, and hyporexia. Yet others present with a waxing and waning course of lesions that spontaneously resolve and recur with a variable response to antimicrobial or subimmunosuppressive courses of systemic corticosteroids. Those having undergone previous excisional biopsies often have a history of dehiscence and/or recurrence of lesions at the surgical site. Pruritus is not a typical feature. Pain occurs more frequently in panniculitis.

Patients with SPDP can be of any breed or sexual status. Patients are often adults; however, the author has observed this syndrome in several dogs between 6 and 12 months of age. Suggested breed predispositions for dermatitis include the golden retriever, boxer, dachshund, collie, Weimaraner, Doberman pinscher, and English bulldog.[1–4] Suggested breed predispositions for panniculitis include poodles,[2,4] dachshunds,[4,5] Australian shepherds,[6] Brittany spaniels,[6] dalmatians,[6] Pomeranians,[6] and Chihuahuas.[6]

Some infectious causes of nodular, pyogranulomatous dermatitis/panniculitis have distinct geographic distributions (**Table 1**). Therefore, travel history and knowledge of regional fungal, bacterial, and oomycotic agents are necessary. Additionally, patients with an active outdoor lifestyle are at higher risk of plant foreign bodies and opportunistic infections associated with puncture wounds (*Actinomyces*, *Sporothrix*) or freshwater activities (*Lagenidium*, *Pythium*).

Patients receiving immunomodulatory drugs, such as prednisolone and cyclosporine (particularly in combination), are more susceptible to opportunistic bacterial and fungal pyogranulomatous infections (**Fig. 1**). *Burkholderia*[7] and bipolaris[8] (phaeohyphomycosis), for example, may be opportunists in such circumstances.

PHYSICAL EXAMINATION

To protect oneself and patients, wear gloves to examine patients with nodular ulcerative dermatoses. Of the infectious differential diagnoses, *Sporothrix* likely has the greatest zoonotic potential. However, opportunistic zoonotic infections may occur with any of the infections mentioned in this text if the skin is broken and direct contact is made, particularly if the handler is immunocompromised. Gloves and proper environmental hygiene may reduce the risk of opportunistic nosocomial staphylococcal infection of ulcerated patients.

SPDP lesions are variable depending on the presence of dermatitis, panniculitis, or both. Regional lymphadenopathy and pyrexia may also be observed. Concurrent sterile pyogranulomatous panniculitis has also been reported in patients with pancreatitis,[9] polyarthritis,[7,10] and systemic lupus erythematosus[11]; thus, abdominal pain, joint pain, or effusion may also be appreciated.

Lesions associated with sterile pyogranulomatous dermatitis include dermal nodules, plaques (**Fig. 2**A), and papules that may ulcerate and drain serous to hemopurulent discharge. Nodules range from 1 cm to 15 cm in size. The lesions may occur

Table 1
Causes of canine pyogranulomatous and granulomatous dermatitis/panniculitis in North America

Cause	Geographic Predilection (if Present)
Foreign body	
Plant material	
Inorganic material	
Inflammatory	
Systemic lupus erythematosus	
Idiopathic vasculitis	
Cutaneous drug eruption, injection reaction	
Sterile arthritis	
Juvenile cellulitis	
Histiocytosis	
Sterile nodular dermatitis/panniculitis	
Infectious	
Pseudomonas (postgrooming furunculosis)	
Burkholderia	
Mycobacterium	
Nocardia	
Actinomyces	
Bartonella	
Cryptococcus	
Sporothrix	
Blastomyces	Mississippi, Missouri, Ohio River Valleys, Mid-Atlantic states, Northeastern Canada
Histoplasma	Mississippi, Missouri, Ohio River Valleys
Coccidioides	Desert Southwest United States, Lower Sonoran Life Zone of Mexico
Pythium	Gulf Coast of United States, US Midwest and Mid-Atlantic states
Lagenidium	Gulf Coast of United States, US Midwest and Mid-Atlantic states
Prototheca	Gulf Coast of United States
Opportunistic fungi (phaeohyphomycosis, hyalohyphomycosis)	
Dermatophytic pseudomycetoma	
Pancreatic	
Neoplasia	
Pancreatitis	

anywhere on the body and are often located on the pinnae, muzzle, periocular regions, and distal extremities.[4]

Lesions associated with sterile pyogranulomatous panniculitis include subcutaneous nodules, ulcers, and draining tracts that may ulcerate and drain oily to hemopurulent discharge (**Fig. 3**). Ulcers may be pinpoint to very large in size and may extend to the muscular layer (**Fig. 3**C and **4**B). Nodules may be firm or fluctuant and involve

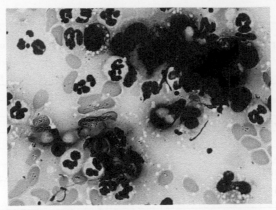

Fig. 1. Fungal hyphae with pyogranulomatous inflammation. Opportunistic infection in dog treated for IMHA (immune mediated hemolytic anemia) with cyclosporine and prednisolone (Romanowsky stain, 100× objective, 1000× total magnification).

the deep dermis as well as the subcutis. Truncal lesions are most common. Scarring may occur following treatment or natural resolution.

Although not well documented, the author has also noted patients with concurrent blepharitis and conjunctivitis (**Fig. 3**A and **4**A). Involvement of the ocular mucous membranes may also be observed with reactive histiocytosis.[2,12] Involvement of the nasal mucous membranes is more typical of reactive histiocytosis.[2,12]

Given the many differential diagnoses associated with nodular and ulcerative pyogranulomatous dermatoses, a thorough physical examination may provide valuable clues to refine differential and diagnostic considerations (eg, aqueous flare and *Blastomyces*).

CONCURRENT DIAGNOSES

Sterile pyogranulomatous dermatitis and panniculitis (SPDP) has been observed with pancreatic neoplasia,[5] polyarthritis,[5,6,10] and systemic lupus erythematosis.[11] An association between sterile pyogranulomatous panniculitis and pancreatitis has been noted in dogs,[9] as it has been in humans.

ETIOPATHOGENESIS

The etiopathogenesis of SPDP is unknown, with no known microbiologic agent or specific antigen stimulus. Prevalence, incidence, and geographic distribution within North America are uncharacterized.

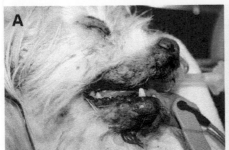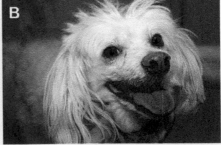

Fig. 2. Poodle mix with plaque form of sterile nodular dermatitis (*A*) and after treatment (*B*).

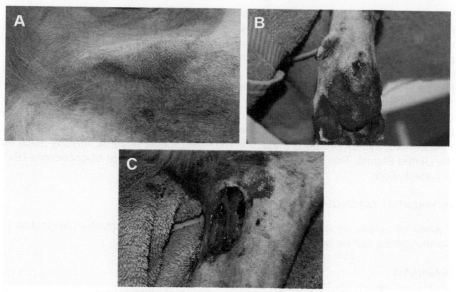

Fig. 3. (*A*) Dermal and subcutaneous nodule on chest of shepherd cross with sterile nodular dermatitis and panniculitis. (*B*) Ulcerated nodule in German shepherd cross. (*C*) Severe ulcerative panniculitis of antebrachium in German shepherd cross.

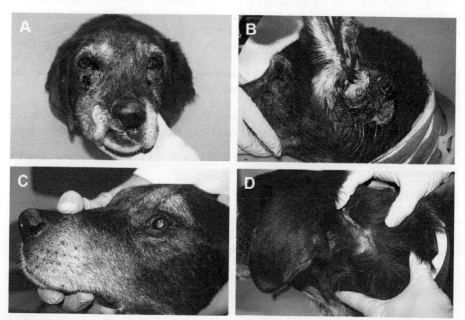

Fig. 4. (*A*) Multiple facial nodules and ulcers with concurrent conjunctivitis and blepharitis, before immunomodulatory treatment. (*B*) Large nodule with ulcer, before immunomodulatory treatment. (*C*) After immunomodulatory therapy. (*D*) Nodule and ulcer resolved after immunomodulatory therapy.

It has been hypothesized that traditional selective bacterial and fungal culture methods may exclude detection of the etiologic agent of SPDP. Next-generation sequence targeting of 16S rRNA and the ITS-1 region of 20 formalin-fixed skin samples and 12 fresh skin samples from dogs diagnosed with sterile granulomatous/pyogranulomatous dermatitis demonstrated no difference in microbiota compared with normal skin samples supporting a sterile cause.[13]

A previous study demonstrated the presence of *Leishmania* DNA in 21 of 46 cases.[14] However, it should be noted that this study investigated dogs in Italy, where *Leishmania* is prevalent; therefore, a strong argument for causation cannot be made. Furthermore, this syndrome is present in non–*Leishmania*-endemic regions (such as the United States). This same study also demonstrated a lack of *Mycobacteria* DNA in these lesions.

DIFFERENTIAL DIAGNOSES

Causes of canine pyogranulomatous and granulomatous dermatitis/panniculitis in North America can be seen in **Table 1**.

DIAGNOSIS

The diagnosis of SPDP is established via exclusion of other causes.

Cytology

Perform multiple cytologic preparations of nodule aspirates, avoiding draining tracts. Review aspirates carefully to assess for the presence of bacterial, fungal, or oomycotic organisms. In infectious cases of pyogranulomatous dermatitis/panniculitis, an etiologic diagnosis may be efficiently made via cytology alone (eg, *Blastomyces*). Cytology of ulcers and draining tracts may reveal secondary infection with cocci and rods, even in SPDP or other sterile processes.

SPDP cytology demonstrates a pyogranulomatous exudate; eosinophils, plasma cells, and lymphocytes may be concurrently present in smaller numbers. Lipid-laden macrophages and free lipid may be observed in panniculitis aspirates. Given severe inflammation, reactive fibrocytes may be seen, leading to misdiagnosis of sarcoma.

Acid-fast stain of aspirates is recommended when *Mycobacterium* is suspected; in some cases poorly staining rods may be visualized in macrophages, and their presence is confirmed via acid-fast stain.

Histopathology

If an etiologic agent is not confirmed via cytology, histopathology is recommended. Biopsy of new lesions is preferable. Avoid draining tracts and ulcers, as they are of poor diagnostic value. Perform multiple biopsies of at least 6 mm in diameter. An excisional wedge is recommended, as the epidermis, dermis, and deep subcutaneous tissues should be included. Request special stains to facilitate the diagnosis of mycobacterial and fungal organisms.

Expected histopathologic findings for SPDP include nodular to diffuse dermal and/or subcutaneous granulomatous or pyogranulomatous dermatitis. In sterile pyogranulomatous dermatitis, the inflammation is often most severe in the peri-adnexal and perivascular areas. Furunculosis as an extension of severe peri-adnexal inflammation may also be present. Lymphocytes, plasma cells, and eosinophils may be present in smaller numbers. Panniculitis may be lobar or septal. Fibrosis is noted in chronic lesions.

Identical histopathologic changes are expected in infectious pyogranulomatous dermatitis and panniculitis. Therefore, histopathologic special stains (Gomori methenamine silver, periodic acid–Schiff, gram, acid fast) and bacterial and fungal cultures are indicated for a definitive diagnosis.

In deep dermal and panniculitis presentations, when neutrophils are less predominant and foamy macrophages are absent, the pathologist may be challenged to distinguish SPDP (macrophages) from histiocytosis (dendritic cells) and rarely nonepitheliotropic lymphoma (poorly differentiated lymphoblasts). Thus, selective immunohistochemical stains, or flow cytometry of tissue aspirates, may be required for diagnosis.

Culture

Collect dermal and subcutaneous tissue samples with an aseptic surgical technique to maximize the yield of the etiologic agent and avoid culture of contaminants. Submit tissue for aerobic and anaerobic bacterial, mycobacterial, and fungal culture. If *Mycobacterium* is suspected, polymerase chain reaction (PCR) may be performed to expedite a definitive diagnosis, as slow-growing *Mycobacterium* species may take several weeks to recover from culture. For the safety of laboratory personnel, fungal culture should be withheld until blastomycosis, coccidioidomycosis, and histoplasmosis have been satisfactorily ruled out via geographic history or a combination of cytology, histopathology, or ancillary diagnostic tests.

Given that opportunistic fungal and bacterial organisms are environmentally ubiquitous (eg, *Alternaria, Burkholderia*), recovery from culture alone, particularly when surface culture is performed instead of tissue culture, is not sufficient for a definitive diagnosis. Cytologic and/or histopathologic evidence for tissue involvement of opportunistic infections is required for a definitive diagnosis.

Patients with SPDP will have negative cultures or culture will yield organisms reflective of secondary bacterial infection of ulcers, frequently *Staphylococcus* sp. Thus, tissue cultures of nonulcerated lesions are recommended.

Additional Tests

Consider complete blood count, serum biochemistry, and urinalysis in patients with systemic clinical signs, such as malaise, pyrexia, hyporexia, abdominal pain, or joint involvement, to assess for pancreatic involvement or evidence for systemic lupus erythematosus. Patients with SPDP alone may have mild, nonregenerative anemia, hyperglobulinemia, and leukocytosis.

Patients with geographic or travel history and signs supportive of blastomycosis, coccidioidomycosis, or histoplasmosis with no organisms found on cytology may be diagnosed via ancillary serologic and urine tests sans fungal culture.

PCR for *Mycobacterium* may confirm or expedite the diagnosis. PCR can be used to distinguish *Pythium* from *Lagenidium* and aid in the diagnosis of these fastidious organisms.

PERPETUATING AND TRIGGERING FACTORS

In the experience of the author, otherwise well-controlled patients receiving immunomodulatory therapy with SPDP may relapse following a triggering immunostimulatory or traumatic event. The author has anecdotally noted generalized relapses associated with vaccination and focal relapses of pyogranulomatous nodular dermatitis in areas of laceration/puncture. These phenomena are not otherwise documented to the author's knowledge.

TREATMENT

Treatment of SPDP involves immunomodulation. A response to systemic corticosteroids is typically rapid when immunosuppressive doses are used. General wound care and ancillary pain management may be required for severe, deep ulcers.

The general treatment strategy involves initiation of clinical remission (**Figs. 2**B and **4**C, D) and attempted maintenance with a nonsteroidal immunomodulatory protocol. The choice of immunomodulator is based on the degree of clinical severity.

For moderate to severe presentations, prednisolone is recommended and a secondary immunomodulator is often added early in therapy as a corticosteroid-sparing or eliminating drug given the delayed time of efficacy for these therapies. Less commonly a secondary immunomodulator is required in conjunction with corticosteroid therapy to induce remission.

In patients with fever, malaise, pain, or advancing disease with no compelling cytologic, physical, or historical evidence of infectious cause, the author will treat patients with prednisone at 0.5 to 1.0 mg/kg by mouth every 24 hours pending confirmation of SPDP via negative culture and supportive histopathology results. Such dosages often provide rapid clinical comfort in SPDP as results await but are insufficient to induce remission in most patients. This relief, of course, must be weighed with the potential risk of worsening infection if an infectious cause is indeed present.

Prednisone/Prednisolone

A total of 2 mg/kg is administered by mouth every 24 hours for initial control for moderate to severe presentations. Lesions typically resolve in 2 to 6 weeks. After this time the dosage can be tapered over a period of 4 to 8 weeks to the lowest every-other-day dosage needed for control with a goal dosage of 0.25 mg/kg every 48 hours, discontinuation, or maintenance with a nonsteroid immunomodulatory.

Doxycycline and Niacinamide

Doxycycline and niacinamide provide well-tolerated immunomodulation for mild cases as a sole therapy or for mild to moderate presentations as a steroid-sparing therapy. This combination may take up to 8 weeks for full effect. Of note, the use of chronic antimicrobial therapy (doxycycline) is considered less favorable in the current era of multidrug-resistant staphylococcal infections.

Niacinamide is administered by mouth every 8 to 12 hours. For dogs less than 10 kg, 250 mg is administered at each dose. For dogs greater than 10 kg, 500 mg is administered at each dose.

Doxycycline is administered at 5.0 to 7.5 mg/kg by mouth twice a day.

Once lesions are resolved, the dosage may be tapered to once daily over a period of a month and, if effective, every-other-day treatment may be attempted.

Cyclosporine (Atopica, Elanco)

A total of 5 to 10 mg/kg is administered by mouth every 24 hours. Cyclosporine provides reliable steroid-sparing control for moderate to severe cases of SPDP and is a reliable sole therapy for mild to moderate presentations. It is important to note that it can take up to 8 weeks for full clinical effect. Once resolution is achieved, the dosage may be reduced to every 48 to 72 hours to maintain resolution.

In the author's experience, cyclosporine is the most reliably effective nonsteroidal immunomodulatory drug for SPDP.

Mycophenolate Mofetil

A total of 20 to 40 mg/kg is administered by mouth divided into 2 or 3 daily dosages. Remission may take up to 8 weeks. This medication has not been well documented as a treatment of SPDP. This medication is better tolerated than azathioprine and is used in moderate to severe cases as a steroid-sparing drug, particularly if cyclosporine is not tolerated.

Azathioprine

A total of 1 to 2 mg/kg by mouth every 24 hours is used for refractory cases or as a steroid-sparing drug. Full clinical effect may take up to 8 weeks. Once remission is achieved, the dosage is reduced to 1 to 2 mg/kg every 48 hours and slowly tapered to the lowest dosage required to maintain remission.

Given the myelotoxic, pancreatic, and hepatotoxic side effects, azathioprine is best reserved for steroid, cyclosporine, and mycophenolate refractory cases. A complete blood count is recommended every 2 weeks as well as serum chemistries for the first 8 weeks of therapy.

Vitamin E

A total of 400 IU every 12 hours is a helpful adjunct antioxidative treatment that has shown to be successful in cases of sterile pyogranulomatous panniculitis.[15]

For solitary lesions, surgical removal may be curative; however, it is possible that new lesions may form. The author has treated cases that have dehisced after surgical removal of the granuloma. The surgery site was infiltrated with pyogranulomatous inflammation.

PROGNOSIS

Prognosis for survival and remission of SPDP is good with immunomodulatory therapy. Scarring may occur and, in the facial area, may result in cicatricial ectropion requiring surgical correction (**Fig. 5**).[3] Most cases require maintenance immunomodulatory therapy to prevent relapse.

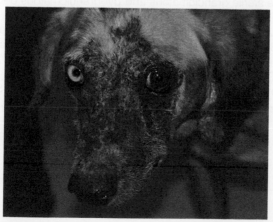

Fig. 5. Cicatricial ectropion in a mixed-breed dog following untreated SPDP.

REFERENCES

1. Panich R, Scott D, Miller W. Canine cutaneous sterile pyogranuloma syndrome: a retrospective analysis of 29 cases (1976-1988). J Am Anim Hosp Assoc 1991;27: 519–28.
2. Gross TL, Ihrke PJ, Walder EJ, et al. Non infectious nodular and diffuse granulomatous and pyogranuloatous diseases of the dermis. Skin diseases of the dog and cat, clinical and histopathologic diagnosis. Ames (IA): Blackwell Science; 2005. p. 320–41.
3. Santoro D, Prisco M, Ciaramella P. Cutaneous sterile granulomas/pyogranulomas, leishmaniasis and mycobacterial infections. J Small Anim Pract 2008; 49(11):552–61.
4. Miller W, Griffin C, Campbell K, et al. Miscellaneous skin diseases In: Muller and Kirk's small animal dermatology. 7th edition. St Louis (MO): Elsevier; 2013. p. 695–719.
5. Yamagishi C, Momoi Y, Kobayashi T, et al. A retrospective study and gene analysis of canine sterile panniculitis. J Vet Med Sci 2007;69:915–24.
6. Contreary CL, Outerbridge CA, Affolter VK, et al. Canine sterile nodular panniculitis: a retrospective study of 39 dogs. Vet Dermatol 2015;26:451–8.
7. Banovic F, Koch S, Robson D, et al. Deep pyoderma caused by Burkholderia cepacia complex associated with ciclosporin administration in dogs: a case series. Vet Dermatol 2015;26(4):287-e64.
8. Rothenburg L, Snider T, Wilson A, et al. Disseminated phaeohyphomycosis in a dog. Med Mycol Case Rep 2017;15:28–32.
9. O'Kell A, Inteeworn N, Diaz SF, et al. Canine sterile nodular panniculitis: a retrospective study of 14 cases. J Vet Intern Med 2010;24:278–84.
10. Gear R, Bacon NJ, Langley-Hobbs S. Panniculitis, polyarthritis, and osteomyelitis associated with pancreatic neoplasia in two dogs. J Small Anim Pract 2006;47: 400–4.
11. Torres S. Sterile nodular dermatitis in dogs. Vet Clin North Am Small Anim Pract 1999;29:1311–4.
12. Miller W, Griffin C, Campbell K, et al. Neoplastic and non-neopastic tumors in: Muller and Kirk's small animal dermatology. 7th edition. St Louis (MO): Elsevier; 2013. p. 818–20.
13. Rosa F, Older C, Meason-Smith C, et al. Analysis of bacterial and fungal nucleic acid in canine sterile granulomatous and pyogranulomatous dermatitis and panniculitis. Vet Pathol 2018;55(1):124–32.
14. Cornegliani L, Fondevila D, Vercelli A, et al. PCR technique detection of *Leishmania* spp. But not *Mycobacterium* spp. in canine cutaneous 'sterile' pyogranuloma/granuloma syndrome. Vet Dermatol 2005;16:233–8.
15. Paterson S. Sterile idiopathic pedal panniculitis in the German shepherd dog – clinical presentation and response to treatment in four cases. J Small Anim Pract 1995;36:498–501.

Canine Cutaneous Lupus Erythematosus
Newly Discovered Variants

Frane Banovic, DVM, PhD

KEYWORDS

• Autoimmune skin disease • Lupus • Skin • Canine • Dermatology

KEY POINTS

• Canine cutaneous lupus erythematosus (CLE) variants are heterogeneous.
• In the generalized form of discoid lupus erythematosus (GDLE) in dogs, erythematous disc-like plaques with adherent scaling and dyspigmentation occur below the neck.
• In mucocutaneous lupus erythematosus (MCLE), erythematous erosions and ulcers affect most commonly anal/perianal regions or genital/perigenital areas in dogs.
• German shepherd dogs and their crosses represent approximately half of the dogs in published MCLE cases.
• Canine GDLE and MCLE seem to respond to a wide range of treatments, but a majority of the cases experience relapse on the tapering of drug dosages.

INTRODUCTION

In humans, the Sontheimer-Gilliam classification divides the skin lesions that can be encountered in lupus erythematosus (LE) into those with characteristic microscopic changes of lymphocyte-rich interface dermatitis with basal keratinocyte damage (ie, lupus-specific skin diseases = cutaneous LE [CLE]) and those without such microscopic pattern (ie, LE-nonspecific skin diseases).[1,2] The LE-specific skin diseases are subdivided into acute CLE, subacute CLE, and chronic CLE (CCLE) types[1]; these designations refer to both the lesional morphology and the average duration of individual skin lesions.[1] Among the several variants of human CCLE (eg, discoid LE [DLE], verrucous (hyperkeratotic) LE, chilblain LE, lupus tumidus, and lupus profundus), DLE represents the most common form.[1,3]

In 1979, Griffin and colleagues[4] reported 2 dogs with localized nasal-predominant dermatitis diagnosed as affected with the canine counterpart of human DLE. Within

The author has nothing to disclose.
Department of Small Animal Medicine and Surgery, College of Veterinary Medicine, University of Georgia, 2200 College Station Road, Athens, GA 30605, USA
E-mail address: fbanovic@uga.edu

Vet Clin Small Anim 49 (2019) 37–45
https://doi.org/10.1016/j.cvsm.2018.08.004
0195-5616/19/Published by Elsevier Inc.

the ensuing 4 decades, novel descriptions of canine CLE variants occurred through several case series.[5–8] Recently, a proposal of the novel CLE classification in dogs (**Fig. 1**), derived from the corresponding human CLE diseases, has been published.[9]

In this review, the author presents the historical and clinical features characteristic of 2 recently described CLE variants, GDLE and mucocutaneous LE (MCLE) and, finally, a review of current treatment recommendations for these variants.

GENERALIZED DISCOID LUPUS ERYTHEMATOSUS
Historical and Clinical Findings

Since the first description of nasal-predominant dermatitis as the canine counterpart of human DLE, 2 large case series of dogs with classic facial (nasal) planum-predominant localized DLE followed (**Fig. 2A**).[10,11] This resulted in the widespread acceptance of canine DLE equated mainly with localized lesions affecting nasal planum. In humans, a distinction between localized DLE, where skin lesions are confined to the head and neck, and the GDLE (GDLE) form, in which skin lesions occur below the neck with or without involvement of the head, exists.[3] Recently, a widespread phenotype that resembled that of the generalized variant of human DLE has been described in dogs.[8,12–14]

Canine GDLE typically affects adult dogs. In a recent case series of 10 dogs, the age of onset of GDLE skin lesions ranged from 5 years to 12 years, with a median age of 9 years.[8] The female/male ratio was 1.0; all dogs were castrated. Different breeds were affected by GDLE (ie, Chinese crested dogs, Labrador retrievers, miniature pinscher, Leonberger, shih tzu, and toy poodle).[8] German shepherd dogs and their crosses, which are predisposed to develop facial (nasal) planum-predominant localized DLE, were not affected by GDLE.[8,9]

The primary lesions in GDLE are annular (discoid) to polycyclic plaques with dyspigmentation (depigmentation and hyperpigmentation), an erythematous margin, adherent scaling, follicular plugging, and central alopecia (**Fig. 2B, C**). The lesions are typically generalized or multifocal and distributed over the neck, dorsum, and lateral and ventral thorax; in some dogs, mucocutaneous junctions are affected. Lesions can advance at clinical presentation; some dogs develop an unusual pattern of diffuse reticulated (netlike) hyperpigmentation whereas in other dogs central atrophic or hypertrophic scars with depigmentation or hyperpigmentation occur (**Fig. 2D–F**).[8]

The main dermatoses with clinical signs mimicking GDLE are hyperkeratotic erythema multiforme and generalized ischemic dermatopathies.[9]

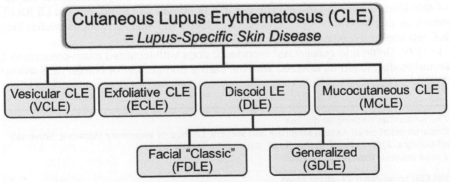

Fig. 1. VCLE, ECLE, localized (facial) DLE or GDLE, and MCLE are the currently recognized subtypes of canine CLE.

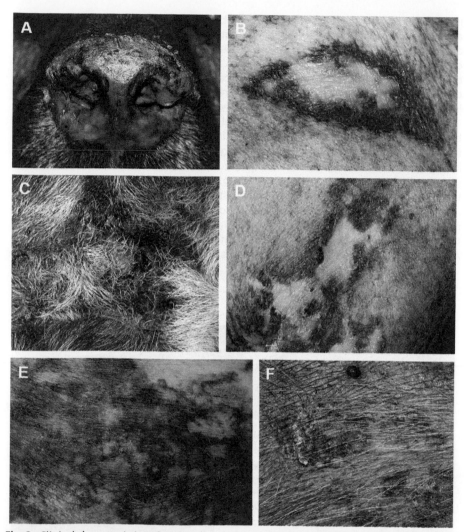

Fig. 2. Clinical characteristics of canine facial and GDLE. (*A*) Erythematous, depigmented, ulcerated, and crusted nasal lesions of facial DLE in a German shepherd dog; complete loss of cobblestone appearance is visible. (*B–D*) Disc-shaped, annular, and polycyclic plaques with hyperpigmentation, focal depigmentation, and scarring on the thorax of dogs with GDLE; foal ulcers at margins are present. (*E*) An unusual pattern of reticulated (netlike) hyperpigmentation with alopecia on the ventral abdomen. (*F*) Hyperpigmented annular macules and patches with central loss of tissue architecture and prominent silver adherent scales surrounded by a peripheral erythematous margin and focal ulceration.

Laboratory, Histopathology, and Immunologic Evaluation

There are no specific routine laboratory findings in canine GDLE. Some human GDLE patients are at risk for development of systemic LE (SLE) within 5 years after the initial diagnosis of skin lesions.[15] The progression to a clinical SLE was observed in only 1 GDLE dog.[16] Despite no clinical signs justifying internal involvement in most GDLE dogs, further investigations, such as complete blood cell count, serum chemistry profile and urinalysis, are performed to rule out concurrent SLE.[8,9] Human SLE patients have high titers of circulating antinuclear antibodies (ANAs); ANAs are autoantibodies against nuclear components, including double-stranded and single-stranded DNA and histones.[15] Therefore, to rule out coexisting SLE, the ANA serology should be evaluated in all dogs diagnosed with GDLE. Although the ANA serology was occasionally positive at a 1:40 serum dilution in the recent GDLE case series, based on the lack of systemic signs and negative laboratory results suggesting renal or hematologic involvement, a diagnosis of coexisting SLE was ruled out in all dogs.[8,9]

Diagnosis of canine GDLE is based on history and clinical presentation supported by characteristic histopathologic findings.[8] Multiple skin biopsies should be collected from affected dogs at the areas of active margin to normal skin. The histology of GDLE in dogs is characterized by a cell-rich, lymphocytic interface dermatitis and folliculitis (Fig. 3A–C).[8] In chronic lesions with scarring, dermal fibrosis occasionally displaces the cell-rich inflammatory infiltrate from the superficial dermis.[8]

Using a direct immunofluorescence method, immunoglobulin deposition at the dermoepidermal junction could be demonstrated in 90% of dogs with GDLE (Fig. 3D)[8]; the deposition resembles the lupus-band test observed in humans with CLE variants. A majority of dogs exhibited a linear deposition of IgG and IgM antibodies at the

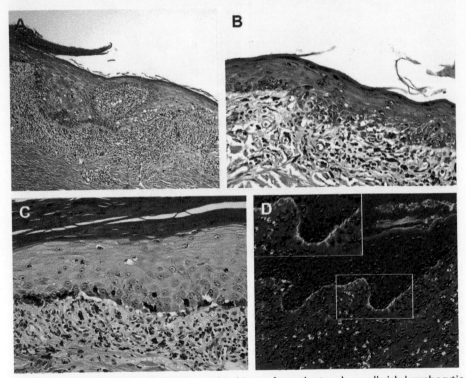

Fig. 3. Histopathology of GDLE. (*A*) In a skin biopsy from the trunk, a cell-rich lymphocytic interface dermatitis is present (H&E, original magnification ×40). (*B, C*) Lymphocytes infiltrate the basal layer of epidermis and are associated with basal cell vacuolation, apoptosis, loss, and disorganization at the cleft margin (H&E, original magnification ×40). (*D*) Continuous and linear IgG deposition along the epidermal basement membrane zone (ie, positive lupus band test). Magnification of IgG deposition with fluorescent round cells in the superficial dermis that represent IgG-positive plasma cells, a common finding at inflamed mucocutaneous junctions (Anti-IgG fluorescein with diamidino phenylindole (DAPI) stain, 109 magnification).

dermoepidermal basement membrane zone of lesional skin, which is similar to what is seen in human DLE lesions.[8]

MUCOCUTANEOUS LUPUS ERYTHEMATOSUS
Historical and Clinical Findings

In the mid-1990s, an erosive skin disease affecting perigenital areas in 2 German shepherd dogs was first reported as a genital-predominant DLE.[17,18] As described previously, chronic juxtamucosal erosive and ulcerative lesions are not a feature of GDLE and facial localized DLE predominantly affects the nasal planum. In 1998, Olivry proposed the diagnosis term, *mucocutaneous LE [MCLE]*, for the canine disease characterized by perimucosal ulcerative lesions areas with a microscopic pathology typical of CLE (Olivry T: British Veterinary Dermatology Study Group, York (United Kingdom), 1998). Unfortunately, the terminology of this canine mucocutaneous disease continued to vary in the past 2 decades; additional cases of similar perimucosal erosive phenotype were published as DLE or perianal/perivulvar LE. In 2015, Olivry and colleagues[7] compared the historical, clinical, and histologic features of 21 dogs affected by erosive mucocutaneous erosions and a CLE histopathology; the MCLE diagnosis was coined for these cases and proposed as another variant of canine CCLE.

MCLE is a rare disease that affects adult dogs of various breeds; German shepherd dogs and their crosses represent approximately half of all published cases of canine MCLE.[7] German shepherd dogs are reported to be predisposed to develop SLE[19–21] and facial localized classic DLE.[10,11] In a case series of 21 dogs, the age of onset of MCLE skin lesions varied widely and ranged from 3 years to 13 years (median; 6 years).[7] The female-to-male ratio was 1.8; if only all published data affecting German/Belgian shepherds and their crosses are included, female dogs appear approximately 4 times over-represented.

One interesting feature of MCLE is that the owners report mucocutaneous sores and pain that manifests while defecating (dyschezia) and/or urinating (dysuria).[7,17,18] The characteristic lesions of MCLE are well-demarcated multifocal to patchy erythematous erosions and ulcers (**Fig. 4**); most cases have symmetric lesions and in some secondary crusting develops. Pigmentary changes, such as hyperpigmentation, often surround ulcerative lesions or develop at the site of previous lesions.[7,17,18]

The mucocutaneous lesions of MCLE most commonly occur on the anal/perianal regions (see **Fig. 4**A) or genital/perigenital (see **Fig. 4**B, C); in rare cases, lesions have been noted around the lips (see **Fig. 4**D), eyes, and nasal planum.[7] At the time of presentation to the veterinarian, a majority of dogs had 2 or more perimucosal or mucocutaneous regions involved.[7] There were no systemic signs observed outside of pain when defecating and urinating or at the site of lesions in the majority of dogs.

Differential diagnoses that can mimic MCLE skin lesions in dogs include mucocutaneous pyoderma (MCP) and mucous membrane pemphigoid (MMP).[7,9] MCP is a poorly characterized skin disease of dogs with greater tendency to affect the nasal planum or the perioral skin, a less erosive and more crusting phenotype, and complete response of lesions to antibiotic therapy.[7,9] MMP affects German shepherd dogs commonly and the skin lesions consist of symmetric erosions/ulcers involving several mucosae and mucocutaneous junctions; histopathology reveals microscopic subepidermal clefts without interface dermatitis characteristic of CLE.[7,9]

Laboratory, Histopathology, and Immunologic Evaluation

There are no specific routine laboratory findings in canine MCLE. Two of 8 patients in a recent case series exhibited very low positive ANA titers without progression to

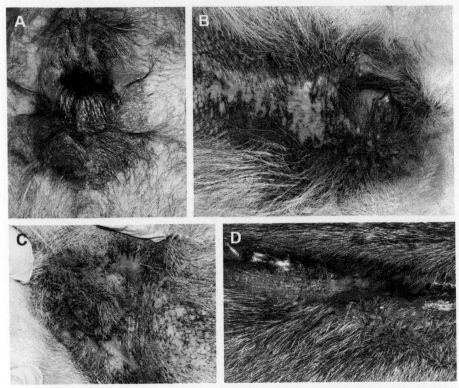

Fig. 4. Clinical characteristics of canine MCLE. (*A*) Anal erosions with peripheral hyperpigmentation in a German shepherd dog; (*B, C*) multifocal genital and perigenital erythematous erosions with peripheral hyperpigmentation are often seen in MCLE lesions; and (*D*) erythematous erosions with crusting at perilabial areas are also seen in MCLE.

SLE.[7] At this time, there is a lack of evidence of signs suggesting an association of canine MCLE with SLE, and the performance of extensive laboratory testing (including ANA serology) in MCLE patients to search for the latter is currently not warranted.[7,9]

Diagnosis of canine MCLE is based on history and clinical presentation supported by characteristic histopathologic findings of cell-rich lymphocytic interface dermatitis with basal keratinocyte damage.[7] Interface dermatitis commonly extends to the infundibula of hair follicles. Multiple biopsies at the margin of the erosions and ulcers are recommended because lymphocytic interface dermatitis in MCLE can be limited to small areas. Not surprisingly, perimucosal erosions and ulcers of MCLE lesions are easily colonized by oral, genital, or fecal bacteria; there is presence of bacterial infection, including neutrophilic crusting and folliculitis in some MCLE skin biopsy sections.[7,9] These findings of secondary surface bacterial colonization or infection may complicate and bias the pathologists because they are suggestive of MCP diagnosis. Therefore, to avoid the presence of infection in MCLE skin biopsies, topical antimicrobials with or without systemic antibiotics are warranted as the first intervention. In MCP cases, complete response to antimicrobial therapy with full remission of lesions is expected to occur.[7,9]

Direct immunofluorescence on paraffin-embedded sections revealed immunoglobulin IgG deposition at the dermoepidermal junction in almost all cases.[7]

TREATMENT AND OUTCOME

The treatment of human CLE variants is divided into nonpharmacologic and pharmacologic approaches; the nonpharmacologic approach is essential and involves photoprotective practices (sun avoidance) through sun-protective clothing along with proper use of sunscreen.[22] Because canine vesicular CLE (VCLE) skin lesions are induced and/or worsened by UV light (ie, frequent lesional flares in summer), sun avoidance is implemented immediately after a diagnosis of VCLE is made.[5,9] Although the exact role of sunlight in the pathogenesis of canine CCLE variants, including GDLE and MCLE, is currently unknown, sun avoidance (keep the dogs out of direct sunlight between 9:00 AM and 5:00 PM) and the use of sunscreen, where possible, is recommended for affected dogs. The American Academy of Dermatology advises the general public to choose a sunscreen with at least sun protection factor (SPF) 50, which protects against UV-B and UV-A, in humans affected by SLE/CLE.[22] Dog sunscreens are available at most pet stores and, similarly to humans, higher SPF is generally recommended.[23]

The pharmacologic therapy approach uses different medications that target some of the key inflammatory pathways involved in the pathogenesis of the CLE disease. The recent 2017 update of the Cochrane systematic review of interventions for human DLE reported evidence for the benefit of a potent topical glucocorticoid; the oral drugs hydroxychloroquine and retinoid acitretin appear to be of equal efficacy in terms of complete resolution in only 50% of patients.[24] The investigators concluded overall low quality and level of reliable evidence and finding the appropriate therapy for a human CLE patient remains challenging.[24] The next challenge is an in-depth understanding of the molecular pathogenesis of human CLE to be able to predict the response of medications in an individual with CLE. Recent insights into the pathogenesis of human CLE at the cellular and molecular levels revealed predominant type 1 helper T-cell (T_H1) lymphocytic inflammatory response with keratinocyte apoptosis and high upregulation of interferon pathway in skin lesions.[25,26] Molecular pathogenesis of canine CLE variants is poorly investigated. Recently, we[27] reported for the first time the lesional skin transcriptome of canine exfoliative CLE (ECLE) variant as well as successful reversal of the skin lesions and associated pathogenic cytokines/chemokines using the oral immunosuppressive medication mycophenolate. The lesional skin of a German shorthaired pointer affected with ECLE expressed strong predominant T_H1 lymphocytic inflammatory response with apoptosis and up-regulation of interferon pathway.[27] Future approaches in the understanding of the molecular pathogenesis of canine GDLE and MCLE skin lesions are warranted to enable the development of specific biomarkers and to evaluate the efficacy of therapeutic strategies at the molecular level.

Skin lesions of canine GDLE and MCLE seem to respond best to immunosuppressive dosages of oral glucocorticoids (1–2 mg/kg prednisone/prednisolone), but a majority of the patients experience relapses on the tapering of drug dosages.[7–9] In a recent retrospective study, the best long-term therapeutic outcome in GDLE skin lesions followed treatment with oral cyclosporine (mean 4.8 mg/kg once daily) along with a short course of glucocorticoids at treatment onset.[8] The treatment modality of oral hydroxychloroquine, in conjunction with topical 0.1% tacrolimus ointment application, helped induce and maintain remission of skin lesions in 2 dogs with GDLE.[8]

Because the erosions and ulcers of MCLE lesions are most commonly localized in perimucosal areas and prone to secondary bacterial colonization or infection, topical antimicrobials with or without systemic antibiotics should be applied in conjunction with immunomodulating treatments for MCLE patients where skin cytology reveals intracellular bacteria and presence of pus.[7] In a majority of cases, oral glucocorticoids induce complete remission of clinical signs within a month of treatment induction.[7,9] Because the tapering of oral glucocorticoids commonly leads to the relapse of MCLE skin lesions, a long-term beneficial response can be achieved using a combination of a tetracycline antibiotic, with or without niacinamide, in some dogs.[7,9] The usefulness of adding topical tacrolimus or additional systemic immunosuppressive drugs (azathioprine, cyclosporine, mycophenolate mofetil, and so forth) for long-term control of MCLE disease should be evaluated further.

SUMMARY

Because the spectrum of canine CLE variants has expanded markedly in the recent 2 decades, veterinarians are encouraged to become familiar with the characteristic clinical features of CLE variants to permit early diagnosis and appropriate treatment. Although the presentations of GDLE and MCLE are clinically distinct, a definitive diagnosis relies on the demonstration of a cell-rich interface dermatitis in skin biopsies taken from affected areas. Skin lesions of canine GDLE and MCLE seem to respond to a wide range of treatments, but half of the cases experienced relapse on the tapering of drug dosages. Sun avoidance is also recommended.

REFERENCES

1. Sontheimer RD. The lexicon of cutaneous lupus erythematosus - A review and personal perspective on the nomenclature and classification of the cutaneous manifestations of lupus erythematosus. Lupus 1997;6:84–95.
2. Kuhn A, Landmann A. The classification and diagnosis of cutaneous lupus erythematosus. J Autoimmun 2014;48-49:14–9.
3. Rothfield N, Sontheimer RD, Bernstein M. Lupus erythematosus: systemic and cutaneous manifestations. Clin Dermatol 2006;24:348–62.
4. Griffin CE, Stannard AA, Ihrke PJ, et al. Canine discoid lupus erythematosus. Vet Immunol Immunopathol 1979;1:79–87.
5. Jackson HA, Olivry T. Ulcerative dermatosis of the Shetland sheepdog and rough colllie dog may represent a novel vesicular variant of cutaneous lupus erythematosus. Vet Dermatol 2001;12:19–28.
6. Bryden SL, Olivry T, White SD, et al. Clinical, histopathological and immunological characteristics of exfoliative cutaneous lupus erythematosus in 25 German short-haired pointers. Vet Dermatol 2005;16:239–52.
7. Olivry T, Rossi MA, Banovic F, et al. Mucocutaneous lupus erythematosus in dogs (21 cases). Vet Dermatol 2015;26:256-e55.
8. Banovic F, Linder KE, Uri M, et al. Clinical and microscopic features of generalized discoid lupus erythematosus in dogs (10 cases). Vet Dermatol 2016;27:488-e131.
9. Olivry T, Linder KE, Banovic F. Cutaneous lupus erythematosus in dogs: a comprehensive review. BMC Vet Res 2018;14(1):132.
10. Scott DW, Walton DK, Manning TO, et al. Canine lupus erythematosus. II. Discoid lupus erythematosus. J Am Hosp Assoc 1983;19:481–8.
11. Olivry T, Alhaidari Z, Carlotti DN, et al. Le lupus érythémateux discoïde du chien: a propos de 22 observations (discoid lupus erythematosus in the dog: 22 cases). Prat Med Chir Anim Comp 1987;22:205–14.

12. Oberkirchner U, Linder KE, Olivry T. Successful treatment of a novel generalized variant of canine discoid lupus erythematosus with oral hydroxychloroquine. Vet Dermatol 2012;23:65–70, e15-6.
13. Banovic F, Olivry T, Linder KE. Ciclosporin therapy for canine generalized discoid lupus erythematosus refractory to doxycycline and niacinamide. Vet Dermatol 2014;25:483-e79.
14. Rossi MA, Messenger LM, Linder KE, et al. Generalized canine discoid lupus erythematosus responsive to tetracycline and niacinamide therapy. J Am Anim Hosp Assoc 2015;51:171–5.
15. Chong BF, Song J, Olsen NJ. Determining risk factors for developing systemic lupus erythematosus in patients with discoid lupus erythematosus. Br J Dermatol 2012;166:29–35.
16. Olivry T, Linder KE. Bilaterally symmetrical alopecia with reticulated hyperpigmentation: a manifestation of cutaneous lupus erythematosus in a dog with systemic lupus erythematosus. Vet Pathol 2013;50:682–5.
17. Poirier N. Discoid lupus erythematosus. Can Vet J 1995;36:493.
18. Bensignor E, Carlotti DN, Pin D. Recto N°38 (perivulvar discoid lupus erythematosus). Prat Med Chir Anim Comp 1997;32:323–4.
19. Hubert B, Teichner M, Fournel C, et al. Spontaneous familial systemic lupus erythematosus in a canine breeding colony. J Comp Pathol 1988;98:81–9.
20. Monier JC, Fournel C, Lapras M, et al. Systemic lupus erythematosus in a colony of dogs. Am J Vet Res 1988;49:46–51.
21. Teichner M, Krumbacher K, Doxiadis I, et al. Systemic lupus erythematosus in dogs: association to the major histocompatibility complex class I antigen DLA-A7. Clin Immunol Immunopathol 1990;55:255–62.
22. Okon LG, Werth VP. Cutaneous lupus erythematosus: diagnosis and treatment. Best Pract Res Clin Rheumatol 2013;27:391–404.
23. Adolph ER, Scott DW, Miller WH, et al. Efficacy of tetracycline and niacinamide for the treatment of cutaneous lupus erythematosus in 17 dogs (1997-2011). Jpn J Vet Dermatol 2014;20:9–15.
24. Jessop S, Whitelaw DA, Grainge MJ, et al. Drugs for discoid lupus erythematosus. Cochrane Database Syst Rev 2017;(5):CD002954.
25. Jabbari A, Suárez-Fariñas M, Fuentes-Duculan J, et al. Dominant Th1 and minimal Th17 skewing in discoid lupus revealed by transcriptomic comparison with psoriasis. J Invest Dermatol 2014;134:87–95.
26. Dey-Rao R, Smith JR, Chow S, et al. Differential gene expression analysis in CCLE lesions provides new insights regarding the genetics basis of skin vs. systemic disease. Genomics 2014;104:144–55.
27. Ferrigno A, Banovic F. Successful treatment of exfoliative cutaneous lupus erythematosus in a German shorthair pointer with mycophenolate mofetil. Abstracts of the North American Veterinary Dermatology Forum May 1–5th 2018, Maui, Hawaii, USA. Vet Dermatol 2018. https://doi.org/10.1111/vde.12546.

Canine Acute Eosinophilic Dermatitis with Edema (Wells-Like Syndrome)

Elizabeth A. Mauldin, DVM

KEYWORDS

- Canine • Eosinophilic dermatitis • Canine Wells-like syndrome
- Sterile neutrophilic dermatitis • Canine Sweet's syndrome

KEY POINTS

- Canine acute eosinophilic dermatitis with edema (CAEDE) is an uncommon syndromic disorder in dogs with a unique clinical presentation.
- Most dogs with CAEDE have a history of gastrointestinal upset preceding or concurrent with onset of skin lesions.
- Dogs with CAEDE present with macular or generalized erythema that is most evident on the glabrous skin of the abdomen.
- Diagnosis of CAEDE is based on clinical and histologic features, but some cases can be difficult to distinguish from canine sterile neutrophilic dermatosis (canine Sweet's syndrome).
- The etiology of CAEDE is not known but an adverse drug reaction or a systemic type I reaction may play a role in the pathogenesis.

INTRODUCTION

Canine acute eosinophilic dermatitis with edema (CAEDE) is an uncommon syndromic disorder in dogs with a unique clinical presentation. Most but not all dogs have a history of moderate to severe gastrointestinal (GI) upset. The skin lesions arise during or after treatment of the GI disease. The affected dogs develop bright red macules or generalized erythema that is most evident on the glabrous skin of the abdomen (**Fig. 1**). The diagnosis is based on both clinical features and histologic features. Although the etiology is not known, adverse drug reaction or unknown systemic hypersensitivity may play a role. Some cases can be difficult to distinguish from canine sterile neutrophilic dermatosis (also known as canine Sweet's syndrome [CSS]) due to overlapping clinical criteria and to eosinophil degranulation in tissue section.

Disclosure Statement: The author has nothing to disclose.
Department of Pathobiology, University of Pennsylvania, School of Veterinary Medicine, 3900 Delancey Street, Philadelphia, PA 19104-6051, USA
E-mail address: emauldin@vet.upenn.edu

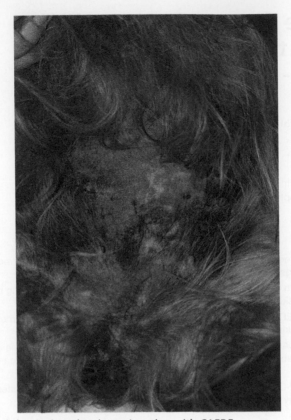

Fig. 1. Marked abdominal erythroderma in a dog with CAEDE.

CLINICAL FEATURES

In 1999, Holm and colleagues[1] published a case series of 9 dogs that presented with an acute onset of erythematous arciform to serpiginous macules and plaques with edema. Skin biopsies revealed a robust eosinophilic inflammatory infiltrate with edema. The syndrome was likened to eosinophilic cellulitis (Wells syndrome) in people.[2] The first dog described in the case series was a Labrador retriever that developed skin lesions while being treated for giardiasis. Holm and colleagues[1] proposed that the skin lesions were triggered by hypersensitivity reaction (eg, drugs or arthropod bites) but definitive causation could not be established.

It is important to differentiate this syndrome from canine atopic dermatitis (CAD). Although dogs with CAD can have acute exacerbations (flares), which may be manifest by generalized erythema, the abrupt onset of the maculopapular lesions along with the histologic features made Holm and colleagues' cases unique. The affected dogs did not have flexural fold or distal extremity lesions (eg, erythema, hyperpigmentation, and lichenification) that define CAD,[3] and pruritus was generally not a feature.[1] And, although CAD is an IgE-mediated disease, histologically, eosinophils are only a minor component of the inflammatory infiltrate.[3,4] The acute dermatitis reported by Holm and colleagues was markedly eosinophilic and some cases had collagen flame figures. Collagen flame figures (ie, foci of densely eosinophilic protein deposits on dermal collagen) are found in intense eosinophilic dermatosis, such as the feline eosinophilic granuloma complex.

A 2006 retrospective study documented an association of the CAEDE syndrome, as described by Holm and colleagues, with GI illness. In that study, 22 of 29 dogs were treated for vomiting and/or diarrhea. Of those, 17 developed skin lesions prior to the GI upset and 5 dogs developed skin lesions concomitantly. Marked diarrhea and vomiting were often accompanied by hematemesis and/or hematochezia and necessitated hospitalization. A majority of dogs were hypoalbuminemic. Like Holm and colleagues' cases, the clinical lesions were consistent: bright red, sometimes targetoid (ie, central clearing) macules, and papules or plaques with or without generalized erythema and edema. The ventral abdominal skin was consistently and most severely affected. A cutaneous drug scoring method was applied to determine the likelihood of an adverse reaction as the etiologic mechanism. Although most dogs received multiple medications (eg, antiemetics, antihistamines, H_2 receptor antagonists, and antibiotics) for the treatment of the GI illness, only 6 dogs with GI disease had a positive drug score. Metronidazole was given to most dogs, but a cause and effect were not proved. In fact, 1 Basset hound whose lesions were believed triggered by metronidazole was unintentionally challenged (given repeated doses) 6 weeks later with no recurrence of skin lesions. Of the 7 dogs without GI illness, 1 dog (a basenji) had a positive drug score. Lesions typical of CAEDE-developed lesions arose while receiving paroxetine for a behavioral problem.[5]

A follow-up study in 2017 by Cain and colleagues[6] investigated those cases of CAEDE with GI illness. As in the prior study, most dogs developed skin lesions after or during treatment of GI distress, but a couple dogs developed the skin lesions 1 day to 2 days prior to the GI upset. Of the 18 dogs, the cause of the GI disorder was identified as pancreatitis in 3 dogs and adverse food reactions in 3 dogs, and 5 dogs were diagnosed with inflammatory bowel disease. A cause for the GI disease was not found in the remaining 8 dogs. Eight dogs had a drug score that was consistent with the possible adverse drug reaction.

Histologically, Cain and colleagues'[6] study showed that the cutaneous inflammation ranged in severity from very mild to severe (**Fig. 2**). The histologic lesion fells into 3 patterns: pattern 1 had very mild eosinophilic with or without neutrophilic inflammation in the superficial dermis with vascular ectasia; pattern 2 had more extensive inflammation that extended into the deeper dermis with few collagen flame figures; and pattern 3 had the most severe and diffuse inflammation.[6] It is important for pathologists to recognize the wide range of inflammation that can occur with CAEDE. The histologic

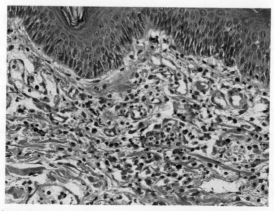

Fig. 2. Moderate dermal eosinophilic inflammatory infiltrate with edema and ectatic blood vessels (*arrows*) (hematoxylin-eosin, original magnification ×10).

lesions likely represent progression of skin lesions, they but do not predict patient outcome or trigger.[6]

ETIOLOGY

Although the pathogenesis of CAEDE remains elusive, the studies by Mauldin and Cain generally refute a similarity of CAEDE with Wells syndrome in people, which tends to be more focal lesion on an extremity.[5,6] The factors common to most canine cases include the following: significant vomiting and diarrhea, which may require hospitalization; hypoproteinemia; treatment with multiple medications; and acute-onset erythroderma and edema in a ventrally oriented distribution. A trigger such as adverse drug reaction may play a role but it is not a definitive cause for all cases. The syndrome is likely a manifestation of systemic type I hypersensitivity reaction.

CLINICAL DIFFERENTIAL DIAGNOSES

Clinically, CAEDE patients develop discrete targetoid (bull's eye) lesions that mimic erythema multiforme and vasculitis. Some dogs may develop pitting edema or facial edema that resembles urticaria. Although vascular damage is histologically evident in many cases (eg, erythrocyte diapediesis and perivascular fibrin accumulation), overt vasculitis (eg, fibrinoid necrosis or leukocytoclasia) is generally not a feature. Furthermore, the skin does not show signs of vascular compromise (cutaneous necrosis or ischemia).[1,5,6] Generally, good-quality skin biopsies can distinguish these conditions.

TREATMENT OF CANINE ACUTE EOSINOPHILIC DERMATITIS WITH EDEMA

In each of the 3 studies on CAEDE, drugs administered prior to the onset of skin lesions were withdrawn.[1,4,6] Commonly administered medications included antiemetics, H_1 and H_2 receptor antagonists, gastroprotectants, anthelmintics, and various antibiotics, including metronidazole. For the skin, medications included corticosteroids (eg, mainly prednisone) and antihistamines (eg, diphenhydramine, cetirizine, and hydroxyzine). The GI disease generally resolved before the skin lesions. In Cain and colleagues'[6] study, GI signs resolved within a week's time whereas the skin lesions took approximately 3 weeks to resolve. The skin lesions typically do not recur. Cain and colleagues[6] reported 1 case of recurrent skin lesions but these occurred without GI signs.[6]

CANINE STERILE NEUTROPHILIC DERMATOSIS (SWEET'S SYNDROME)

Sterile neutrophilic dermatosis (CSS) is a rare disorder with features that overlap CAEDE. This condition has been equated to acute febrile neutrophilic dermatosis (also known as Sweet's syndrome) in people. Dogs and humans with Sweet's syndrome may show signs of systemic illness (eg, fever, neutrophilia, arthritis, or pneumonia).[7–11] In dogs, skin lesions are similar but perhaps more pustular than CAEDE and also may be most apparent on glabrous skin. Histologically, the dermis contains a marked neutrophilic infiltrate with or without eosinophils. Some cases have been putatively associated with adverse drug reactions.[10,11]

CASES OF OVERLAPPING CANINE ACUTE EOSINOPHILIC DERMATITIS WITH EDEMA AND CANINE SWEET'S SYNDROME

Clinical lesions and histologic features may overlap in cases of CAEDE and CSS. There are 3 main reasons why the diagnosis can be challenging: (1) eosinophils in tissue section may undergo degranulation, thus making it difficult to distinguish them from neutrophils; (2) eosinophils have been reported as a component of the inflammatory infiltrate in CSS; and (3) some cases in the older literature of diagnosis as CSS might now be classified as CAEDE. Indeed, sterile pustular erythroderma of miniature schnauzers is a condition whose histologic features can be identical to either CAEDE or CSS depending on whether neutrophils or eosinophils predominate in the dermal inflammatory infiltrate.[12] Miniature schnauzers were represented in the CAEDE Mauldin and Cain and colleagues' studies.[5,6] It is possible that these disorders are interrelated and represent of broad spectrum of systemic hypersensitivity with skin manifestations. For pathologists who have difficulty in distinguishing the granulocytes in tissue section, a Luna histochemical stain can be applied to assess for the granules in eosinophils.[13]

REFERENCES

1. Holm KS, Morris DO, Gomez SM, et al. Eosinophilic dermatitis with edema in nine dogs, compared with eosinophilic cellulitis in humans. J Am Vet Med Assoc 1999; 215(5):649–53.

2. Wells G, Smith NP. Eosinophilic cellulitis. Br J Dermatol 1979;100:101–9.

3. Olivry T, Hill PB. The ACVD task force on canine atopic dermatitis(XVIII): histopathology of skin lesions. Vet Immunol Immunopathol 2001;81:305–9.

4. Bizikova P, Santaro D, Marsella R, et al. Review: clinical and histological manifestations of canine atopic dermatitis. Vet Dermatol 2015;26:79-e24.

5. Mauldin EA, Palmeiro BS, Goldschmidt MH, et al. Comparison of clinical history and dermatologic findings in 29 dogs with severe eosinophilic dermatitis: a retrospective analysis. Vet Dermatol 2006;17(5):338–47.

6. Cain CL, Bradley CW 2nd, Mauldin EA. Clinical and histologic features of acute-onset erythroderma in dogs with gastrointestinal disease: 18 cases (2005-2015). J Am Vet Med Assoc 2017;251(12):1439–49.

7. Gains MJ, Morency A, Sauve F, et al. Canine sterile neutrophilic dermatitis (resembling Sweet's syndrome) in a Dachshund. Can Vet J 2010;51(12):1397–9.

8. Johnson CS, May ER, Myers RK, et al. Extracutaneous neutrophilic inflammation in a dog with lesions resembling Sweet's Syndrome. Vet Dermatol 2009;20(3): 200–5.

9. Cohen PR, Kurzrock R. Sweet's syndrome revisited: a review of disease concepts. Int J Dermatol 2003;42(10):761–78.

10. Mellor PJ, Roulois AJ, Day MJ, et al. Neutrophilic dermatitis and immune-mediated haematological disorders in a dog: suspected adverse reaction to carprofen. J Small Anim Pract 2005;46(5):237–42.

11. Vitale CB, Ihrke PJ, Gross TL. Putative diethylcarbamazine-induced urticaria with eosinophilic dermatitis in a dog. Vet Dermatol 1994;5(4):197–203.

12. Okada K, Saegusa S, Yamaoka A, et al. Febrile neutrophilic dermatosis in a miniature schnauzer resembling Sweet's syndrome in humans. Vet Dermatol 2004; 15(s1).

13. Gomes P, Torres SM, Plager DA, et al. Comparison of three staining methods to identify eosinophils in formalin-fixed canine skin. Vet Dermatol 2013;24(3):323–8, e71–2.

Canine Perianal Fistulas
Clinical Presentation, Pathogenesis, and Management

Christine L. Cain, DVM

KEYWORDS

- Canine • Perianal fistula • Anal furunculosis • German shepherd dog
- Immune-mediated • Cyclosporin A

KEY POINTS

- Canine perianal fistulas are painful ulcers or sinus tracts that spontaneously occur in the skin around the anus and can be debilitating for affected dogs.
- Middle-aged German shepherd dogs are most commonly affected and may have a genetic susceptibility, but other purebred and mixed-breed dogs also develop perianal fistulas.
- Although anatomic factors were once believed to contribute to development, an immune-mediated pathogenesis is now recognized.
- Over the years, there has been a paradigm shift from surgical management to long-term medical management of canine perianal fistulas.
- Immunomodulatory medications, in particular cyclosporin A with or without ketoconazole, are most commonly used for management of canine perianal fistulas.

INTRODUCTION

Perianal fistulas, also known as anal furunculosis, are painful sinus tracts or ulcers that spontaneously occur in the skin around the anus (**Fig. 1**). German shepherd dogs are predisposed to developing perianal fistulas, but other purebred and mixed-breed dogs also are affected. Although development of perianal fistulas was once believed related to anatomic conformation, the condition is now recognized as immune mediated, although the pathogenesis has not been fully delineated. Likewise, although surgical intervention and correction of anatomic factors were once the mainstays of therapy, medical management is the current standard of care for dogs with perianal fistulas. This condition can be debilitating for affected dogs and can result in

Disclosure Statement: The author has nothing to disclose.
Dermatology, Department of Clinical Sciences and Advanced Medicine, University of Pennsylvania, School of Veterinary Medicine, 3900 Delancey Street, Room 2065, Philadelphia, PA 19104, USA
E-mail address: ccain@vet.upenn.edu

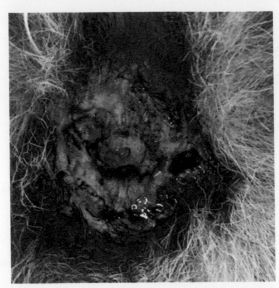

Fig. 1. Multiple sinus tracts around the anus in a 7-year-old intact male German shepherd dog.

euthanasia if not effectively managed. Rapid and accurate diagnosis and aggressive medical therapy are key to successful management of canine perianal fistulas. This article reviews current knowledge regarding the clinical presentation, pathogenesis, and medical management of perianal fistulas.

CLINICAL PRESENTATION

Dogs with perianal fistulas may present with a single or multiple sinus tracts or ulcers in the skin around the anus. In some cases, ulcers may be large and deep or crateriform. Despite widespread use of the term, *perianal fistula*, in the veterinary medical literature, the cutaneous sinus tracts do not generally communicate with the rectal lumen (as is the case for humans with fistulizing Crohn's disease).[1] Due to the location and discomfort on examination, dog owners may not be aware of the lesions but may present their dog to the veterinarian due to associated clinical signs, such as licking around the anus, tenesmus, hematochezia, or mucopurulent discharge (**Fig. 2**).[2,3] An association between perianal fistulas and colitis has been demonstrated, and some affected dogs also may have a history of soft or mucoid stools, diarrhea, and increased frequency of defecation.[2,3]

German shepherd dogs are most commonly affected (reported to comprise more than 80% of the patient population[4]), but several other breeds, including the beagle, border collie, Australian shepherd, Irish setter, Chesapeake Bay retriever, Leonberger, Staffordshire bull terrier, and mixed-breed dogs, have also been reported to develop perianal fistulas.[3–10] The author has also diagnosed perianal fistulas in an American Staffordshire terrier (**Fig. 3**), a Brittany spaniel, a soft-coated wheaten terrier, and mixed-breed dogs.

Perianal fistulas are typically adult onset. The age of onset can vary widely, from young adult to geriatric, although middle-aged dogs are most commonly affected.[4,5,11] A definitive gender predisposition has not been demonstrated, although

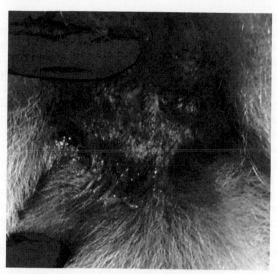

Fig. 2. Perianal ulcer with mucopurulent exudate in an 8-year-old intact male German shepherd dog. This dog also presented with severe tenesmus.

an increased risk in intact male German shepherd dogs compared with neutered male German shepherd dogs has been suggested.[12]

DIAGNOSIS

Perianal fistulas are visually distinct and, in most cases, are diagnosed based on clinical presentation alone, especially in a German shepherd dog. An ulcerated perianal neoplasm (perianal adenoma or adenocarcinoma) and mucocutaneous lupus

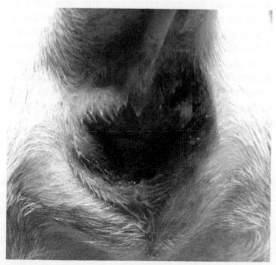

Fig. 3. Multiple perianal ulcers and sinus tracts in 6-year-old castrated male American Staffordshire terrier dog. This dog also had a history of chronic diarrhea and inflammatory bowel disease (colitis and proctitis) confirmed via endoscopic biopsies.

erythematosus (MCLE) are the primary rule-outs, but other conditions resulting in peri-anal draining tracts also should be considered. For example, glandular tissue left behind after an anal sacculectomy can result in chronic perianal draining tracts that can be misdiagnosed as perianal fistulas. German shepherd dogs are also predis-posed to MCLE, and anal or perianal lesions are common in this condition.[13] Perianal fistulas generally are clinically differentiated from MCLE. Perianal fistulas are typically sharply demarcated sinus tracts or crateriform ulcers, whereas MCLE is associated with more confluent erosions, ulcers, erythema, and crusts.[13] For more information about canine MCLE, see Frane Banovic's article, "Canine Cutaneous Lupus Erythematosus Newly Discovered Variants," in this issue.

Histopathology is rarely performed for diagnosis of canine perianal fistulas but can be considered in cases of unusual clinical presentation or in an uncommonly affected breed (such as a small breed dog). In humans with perianal fistulas due to Crohn's dis-ease, malignant transformation can occur and, although not well documented in dogs with perianal fistulas, could be a reason to prioritize histopathology in patients with chronic disease.[14]

Histopathologic features of canine perianal fistulas include periadnexal inflamma-tion with or without furunculosis, pronounced hidradenitis, periadnexal fibrosis, ulcer-ation, and formation of epithelial-lined sinus tracts within the dermis.[4,5] Inflammatory infiltrates, composed of neutrophils, lymphocytes, plasma cells, and macrophages, may be noted within sinus tracts.[4] Deeper lesions also may be associated with pyog-ranulomatous cellulitis and lymphoid follicles.[5] If clinical differentiation of perianal fis-tulas from MCLE is difficult, skin biopsies for histopathology may be helpful. MCLE is characterized by a lymphocyte-rich interface dermatitis with evidence of basal cell damage.[13] Colonic biopsies from dogs with perianal fistulas may demonstrate histo-pathologic evidence of colitis; 1 study found histopathologic changes consistent with a diagnosis of colitis in 9 of 18 dogs with perianal fistulas.[3]

In addition to close examination of the perianal skin, the physical examination for dogs suspected of having perianal fistulas should include a rectal examination. Seda-tion may be required to accomplish this and is dependent on patient comfort level. All patients should be assessed for anal strictures, the anal sacs should be carefully palpated, and expression of the anal sacs should be attempted. Abnormalities of the anal sacs, including impaction, difficult expression, or rupture, may occur in pa-tients with perianal fistulas and are usually secondary to inflammation and fibrosis in the region of the anal sac ducts.[15,16] The author has encountered perianal fistulas and a concurrent apocrine gland adenocarcinoma of the anal sac in the same patient (a middle-aged German shepherd dog). This patient presented with a mildly enlarged, firm, and nonexpressible anal sac that did not markedly change despite resolution of the perianal fistulas with medical therapy.

PATHOGENESIS

The predisposition to development of perianal fistulas in German shepherd dogs was initially believed related to anatomic conformation. Several conformational features were speculated to contribute to the development of perianal fistulas, including low tail carriage encouraging fecal retention and an increased density of perianal apocrine sweat glands.[5,11] The low tail carriage was believed to produce a warm, humid envi-ronment, leading to chronic inflammation and secondary infection of perianal and anal glands with fecal flora.[11] The occurrence of perianal fistulas in other dog breeds without low tail carriage, as well as the lack of a clinical response to antimicrobial ther-apy alone, led investigators to question this anatomic conformation theory.[5]

Gradually, a probable immune-mediated pathogenesis for canine perianal fistulas emerged. An early study investigating the immunologic status of dogs with perianal fistulas demonstrated a blunted lymphocyte proliferation response following stimulation with phytomitogens in 9 of 33 dogs with active disease. After lesion resolution, the lymphocyte proliferation response normalized in 4 of 9 dogs. Based on this result, the investigators suggested that the suppression of the lymphocyte proliferation response may be an acquired abnormality secondary to perianal fistulas.[17] More recent work has demonstrated that perianal fistulas likely develop as a consequence of local T-cell–mediated inflammation. This is supported by studies demonstrating perivascular aggregates of CD3[+] T lymphocytes within lesional skin of dogs with perianal fistulas[18] as well as increased expression of T-cell–associated, in particular type 1 helper T-cell–associated cytokine mRNA in lesional skin of affected dogs compared with controls.[6] A decrease in expression of interleukin (IL)-2 in lesional skin after cyclosporin A therapy has also been demonstrated.[8] Abnormal macrophage activation by type 1 helper T cells has also been suggested to play a role in the development of perianal fistulas. One study found increased expression of matrix metalloproteinase (MMP)-9 and MMP-13 mRNA in lesional skin from dogs with perianal fistulas compared with controls. MMP-9 and MMP-13 are produced by activated macrophages and are involved in the early stages of wound healing, primarily by degradation of the extracellular matrix. The investigators of this study proposed that impaired wound healing, in particular failure to initiate wound repair, may play a role in the persistence of ulcers and sinus tracts.[7] Similarly, up-regulation of MMPs may play a role in the pathogenesis of human fistulizing Crohn's disease, which is proposed to be a correlate of canine perianal fistulas.[19]

A dysfunctional immune response to microbes in the anal and perianal regions also has been proposed to contribute to the pathogenesis of canine perianal fistulas. One culture-based study performed in 1988 from tissue samples collected at the time of surgical fistula excision showed that Escherichia coli, Staphylococcus sp, β-hemolytic streptococci, and Proteus mirabilis were isolated most frequently. The investigators concluded that the bacterial isolates likely represented contaminants and that microbial infection did not play a primary role in the development of perianal fistulas.[5] In 2008, House and colleagues[20] investigated mRNA expression and function of several pattern recognition receptors in vitro using monocyte/macrophages derived from the blood of dogs with perianal fistulas. They found evidence of a decreased response in the NOD2 pattern recognition receptor of macrophage/monocytes derived from dogs with perianal fistulas after stimulation with microbial pathogen-associated molecular patterns compared with controls. This result suggests a possible innate immunodeficiency in dogs with perianal fistulas. Dogs with perianal fistulas were also shown to have increased antistaphylococcal IgG compared with normal dogs[21] and a dysregulated T-cell–mediated response to cutaneous or fecal microbial antigens in dogs with perianal fistulas has been proposed.[8]

Since these studies were performed in the late 1990s and early 2000s, there has been an increasing focus in the medical community on characterization of microbial populations (the microbiome) via non–culture-based methods and on the complex interplay between shifts in microbial populations and the promotion of disease. Shifts in the cutaneous and/or intestinal microbiome have been proposed to contribute to the development of hidradenitis suppurativa (also proposed as a human correlate of canine perianal fistulas), although this link has not been well established.[22] Intestinal dysbiosis has been well described in association with inflammatory bowel disease in humans,[23] and manipulation of the intestinal microbial flora via fecal transplantation may be effective at ameliorating the clinical signs of Crohn's disease and ulcerative colitis in humans.[24] To explore the role that cutaneous and intestinal microbial populations may play in canine perianal fistulas, the author and colleagues have completed a longitudinal evaluation of the cutaneous and rectal microbiome in German shepherd dogs with perianal fistulas, both prior to and while receiving immunomodulatory therapy with cyclosporin A and ketoconazole (the study was funded by an internal grant from the Penn Vet Center for Host-Microbial Interactions, Philadelphia, Pennsylvania). Clinically normal German shepherd dogs were sampled as a control population; data analysis currently is in progress.

An adverse food reaction has been reported for some dogs with perianal fistulas. One study of adverse food reactions in dogs with dermatologic signs reported a significant association between perianal fistulas and adverse food reaction, but only 4 dogs with perianal fistulas were included and all were German shepherd dogs.[25] Three studies reported a positive clinical response to a novel protein diet in dogs with perianal fistulas; in 1 study, a fish and potato diet was fed long term after surgical excision of sinus tracts and bilateral anal sacculectomy.[9] In the second study, dogs were fed an exclusive venison and potato or fish and potato diet but also received metronidazole initially as well as topical tacrolimus 0.1% ointment and a tapering course of oral prednisone for 16 weeks.[26] In the third study, dogs were fed a commercially available lamb and rice or vegetarian diet but concurrently received a tapering course of oral prednisone at an initial immunosuppressive dose.[2] Although the author regularly recommends an elimination diet trial using a prescription novel protein or hydrolyzed protein diet as part of the diagnostic work-up for dogs with perianal fistulas, it is unclear from the available literature how many dogs may achieve long-term disease remission with dietary control alone.

GENETIC BASIS

The strong association of perianal fistulas with the German shepherd breed suggests a genetic susceptibility. A few studies have explored potential genetic risk factors for the disease in German shepherd dogs. An association between the class II MHC allele DLA-DRB1*00101 and increased risk of development of perianal fistulas has been found in populations of German shepherd dogs from the United Kingdom and Finland. Dogs homozygous for the DLA-DRB1*00101 allele may develop perianal fistulas earlier in life (at <8 years of age).[12,27] Class II molecules of the major histocompatibility complex (MHC) are involved in antigen presentation and T-cell activation; thus, an association with an MHC allele further supports a T-cell–mediated pathogenesis for this disease.[12,27] A genome-wide association study of 21 affected German shepherd dogs and 25 unaffected German shepherd dogs, followed by genotyping of potentially associated single nucleotide polymorphisms in cohorts of affected and unaffected German shepherd dogs in the United Kingdom and Finland, found a potential association with the ADAMTS16 and CTNND2 gene regions.[28] The CTNND2 gene region also has been associated with human Crohn's disease and ulcerative colitis, suggesting a potential shared pathogenesis for human inflammatory bowel disease and canine perianal fistulas.[28] Another study investigated genes encoding for several pattern recognition receptors in German shepherd dogs with perianal fistulas. This study failed to identify any single nucleotide polymorphisms in genes encoding for pattern recognition receptors associated with perianal fistulas but did show restricted pattern recognition receptor genotypes in German shepherd dogs (both affected and unaffected) versus other dog breeds. The restricted pattern recognition receptor genotypes in German shepherd dogs may influence innate immune function in this breed.[29]

HUMAN CORRELATES

Two human conditions, hidradenitis suppurativa and fistulizing Crohn's disease, have been proposed as correlates of canine perianal fistulas.[5,10] Like perianal fistulas in dogs, both of these conditions are painful and debilitating and can have a negative impact on quality of life of patients.[19,22,30] Management of both of these conditions is challenging: no universally effective therapy has been identified and relapses are common.[14,19,22,30]

Hidradenitis suppurativa is associated with nodules, abscesses, sinus tracts, and scarring, primarily in intertriginous regions (axilla, groin, perianal region, and mammary region).[22] Hidradenitis suppurativa was initially proposed as a potential correlate of canine perianal fistulas because of similar histopathologic features, including furunculosis, hidradenitis, and formation of epithelial-lined sinus tracts.[5,22] The pathogenesis of hidradenitis suppurativa has not been fully elucidated, but it is likely an immune-mediated condition with a genetic susceptibility. Alterations in cutaneous or intestinal microbiota may play a role in the pathogenesis. Risk factors include obesity, smoking, metabolic syndrome, hormonal influences, and diabetes mellitus; an association with inflammatory bowel disease has also been suggested.[22,31] Medical management of hidradenitis suppurativa involves use of topical or systemic antimicrobials (potentially helpful for anti-inflammatory and/or immunomodulatory properties more so than direct targeting of microbes), retinoids, systemic or intralesional corticosteroids, and cytokine-directed therapies (inhibitors of tumor necrosis factor [TNF] or IL-1).[30]

Perianal manifestations of Crohn's disease are common, estimated to affect 25% to 33% of Crohn's disease patients.[14,19,32] Perianal fistulas are more common in patients with colonic or rectal disease and may be simple (a fistulous tract with a single external opening) or complex (multiple fistulous tracts, perianal abscesses, or anal/rectal stricture).[14,19] Unlike the typical disease in dogs, these are true fistulas that communicate with the intestinal lumen. The pathogenesis of perianal fistulas in Crohn's disease is not fully understood but has been shown to involve epithelial-to-mesenchymal transition and up-regulation of MMPs and proinflammatory cytokines. Genetic susceptibility, as well as alterations in the cutaneous and/or intestinal microbiota, may play a role in development of perianal fistulas in humans.[14,19] Like canine perianal fistulas, there has been a shift in management of fistulizing Crohn's disease from primarily surgical intervention to incorporation of medical therapies.[32] Successful management of fistulizing Crohn's disease usually necessitates multimodal surgical and medical approaches. To date, the most efficacious medical therapies are cytokine-directed therapies (inhibitors of TNF or IL-12/IL-23), intrafistula mesenchymal stem cell injections, and adjunctive antimicrobials (although antimicrobials alone are not effective for resolution of fistulas).[1,14,19,32]

Both hidradenitis suppurativa and fistulizing Crohn's disease share clinical features with canine perianal fistulas. Similarities in the pathogenesis of hidradenitis suppurativa and Crohn's disease have been demonstrated, in particular infiltration of diseased tissue by type 17 T helper cells.[33] Future studies should focus on better characterization of the underlying etiology of these 3 conditions and may help direct the development of future therapies, such as antibodies targeting specific cytokines, for perianal fistulas in dogs.

SURGICAL MANAGEMENT

A comprehensive review of surgical management of canine perianal fistulas is beyond the scope of this article. With the increasing recognition of an immune-mediated pathogenesis for the disease, there was a corresponding shift in standard-of-care from surgical intervention to medical management. Several surgical procedures have been described, including en bloc surgical excision (usually performed together with bilateral anal sacculectomy) followed by surgical reconstruction, laser excision, cryosurgery, and amputation at the tail base.[9,15,16,34–37] One study reported good control of perianal fistulas using a combination of immunomodulatory therapy with prednisone and azathioprine or cyclosporin A with or without ketoconazole followed by surgical excision of remaining sinus tracts, bilateral anal sacculectomy, and cryptectomy.[35] Another study reported a complete response (lack of visible sinus tracts or ulcers) in 29 of 33 dogs after en bloc surgical resection of perianal fistulas, bilateral anal sacculectomy, and diet change to a fish and potato diet. Six of these 29 dogs continued to exhibit clinical signs, such as perianal licking, tenesmus, diarrhea, or constipation.[9] Potential complications of surgical repair of perianal fistulas include dehiscence, lesion recurrence (reported in more than 50% of dogs in one study[34]), likely related to the failure to control the underlying immune-mediated inflammation, fecal incontinence, and anal stricture.[16,34]

MEDICAL MANAGEMENT
Mesenchymal Stem Cell Injections

Injections of mesenchymal stem cells, administered directly into fistulas, have been shown effective for humans with fistulizing Crohn's disease.[1] Mesenchymal stem cells have immunomodulatory activity, such as decreasing proliferation and activation of T lymphocytes and dendritic cells and increasing production of T-regulatory cells.[10,19] The efficacy of mesenchymal stem cell injections for canine perianal fistulas has been reported for a small number of dogs by Ferrer and colleagues.[10] Six dogs with perianal fistulas that had failed therapy with cyclosporin A at standard dosing for a minimum of 6 months of administration were enrolled in an open-label trial and received a single injection of human embryonic stem cell–derived mesenchymal stem cells within perianal lesions. The dogs were followed for 6 months postinjection; all dogs had resolution of sinus tracts or ulcers by 3 months after injection of stem cells. Two dogs had recurrence of perianal fistulas by 6 months postinjection.[10] Although mesenchymal stem cell injections are a promising treatment option for canine perianal fistulas, additional controlled studies are needed to apply these results to larger populations of affected dogs as well as to determine the optimal frequency of injections.

Antimicrobials

Antimicrobials alone do not seem effective for management of perianal fistulas in dogs. In the author's experience, many dogs are treated with antimicrobials at the time of onset of clinical signs of perianal fistulas but continue to experience disease progression. A few studies have reported use of metronidazole in combination with other therapies (azathioprine, tacrolimus ointment, prednisone, and novel protein diet) for treatment of dogs with perianal fistulas.[26,38] In addition to activity against anaerobic bacteria and protozoa, metronidazole may also have anti-inflammatory activity, including promotion of T-regulatory cell differentiation.[39] This anti-inflammatory activity may aid in treatment of immune-mediated diseases, but the efficacy of metronidazole alone for treatment of perianal fistulas is unknown at this time.

Immunomodulatory Agents

Several immunomodulatory agents have been reported as treatments for canine perianal fistulas, including oral prednisone (at initial immunosuppressive doses), azathioprine, cyclosporin A (alone or in combination with ketoconazole), topical tacrolimus, and mycophenolate mofetil.[2,35,38,40–51] The best evidence of efficacy is for calcineurin inhibitors (cyclosporin A and tacrolimus); these are discussed later. In 1 study of German shepherd dogs with perianal fistulas treated with a tapering course of oral prednisone (at an initial immunosuppressive dose of 2 mg/kg/d) and a commercially available novel protein diet for up to16 weeks, complete lesion resolution was noted in 9 of 27 dogs (33.3%).[2] Due to the need for ongoing administration of immunomodulatory agents for management, as well as the risk of side effects with long-term administration of corticosteroids, the author does not typically use corticosteroids for management of canine perianal fistulas. In another study by Harkin and colleagues,[40] 14 dogs with perianal fistulas were treated with azathioprine alone. After 16 weeks of therapy, 8 of 14 dogs (57%) achieved complete resolution of lesions. To the author's knowledge, there is only a single report of the use of mycophenolate mofetil for the management of perianal fistulas in the veterinary literature; this dog was treated for 4 weeks without improvement in lesions.[51]

Calcineurin Inhibitors (Cyclosporin A and Tacrolimus)

Cyclosporin A and tacrolimus are immunomodulatory agents that work by binding to the intracellular protein cyclophilin-1, which inhibits calcineurin. This inhibition of calcineurin prevents the dephosphorylation of nuclear factor of activated T cells and subsequent production of proinflammatory cytokines, such as IL-2. Decreased production of IL-2 leads to decreased growth and activation of T lymphocytes.[52]

Several studies have supported the efficacy of cyclosporin A for treatment of canine perianal fistulas, including randomized and controlled clinical trials. In a randomized clinical trial comparing cyclosporin A with a placebo in German shepherd dogs with perianal fistulas, complete lesion resolution was reported in 17 of 20 dogs (85%) receiving cyclosporin A after 16 weeks of treatment. Mean total surface area and depth of lesions improved by 78% and 62%, respectively, after 4 weeks of therapy in dogs receiving cyclosporin A.[41]

Cyclosporin A doses investigated for treatment of canine perianal fistulas vary widely—from 1.5 mg/kg every 24 hours to 10 mg/kg every 12 hours.[42–46] In general, higher doses were associated with improved outcome,[46] but all dogs were not treated with the same formulation of cyclosporin A (some received nonmodified cyclosporin A)[42] and cyclosporin A was administered with food in some cases.[43] Modified or microemulsified formulations of cyclosporin A have superior bioavailability in dogs and should be used preferentially in all cases. Bioavailability of cyclosporin A in dogs is also reduced by the presence of food and it is best administered on an empty stomach (ie, 2 hours prior to or after a meal).[52]

The cost of cyclosporin A, particularly at higher doses or for larger dogs, may be prohibitive. Administration of cyclosporin A with ketoconazole can inhibit metabolism of cyclosporin A by hepatic cytochrome P450 microenzymes as well as improve bioavailability via inhibition of intestinal P-glycoprotein (thus decreasing transport of cyclosporin A to the intestinal lumen). Coadministration of the 2 drugs can improve cyclosporin A bioavailability by 75% or more, depending on the ketoconazole dose, and allow cyclosporin A dose reduction.[47,52] The combination of cyclosporin A (at doses of 1 mg/kg/d to 5.5 mg/kg/d) and ketoconazole (at doses of 5.1 mg/kg/d to 11 mg/kg/d) was shown effective in clinical trials with complete lesion resolution in 93% of dogs in 16 weeks,[48] 100% of dogs in 3 to 10 weeks,[49] and 67% of dogs with a mean time to resolution of 13.9 weeks.[47]

The author regularly uses the combination of cyclosporin A at initial doses of 2 mg/kg/d to 4 mg/kg/d and ketoconazole at initial doses of 5 mg/kg/d to 10 mg/kg/d for treating perianal fistulas in dogs. Relapses can occur when immunomodulatory therapy is discontinued.[41,43,45–49] For this reason, after complete resolution of lesions (which generally requires 8–12 weeks of therapy), the author slowly tapers cyclosporin A and ketoconazole to the lowest effective dosing and dose frequency. The author does not routinely perform cyclosporin A blood level monitoring in these patients because cyclosporin A blood levels do not correlate well with clinical response.[46]

Tacrolimus 0.1% ointment has also been shown effective for treatment of canine perianal fistulas, although randomized controlled clinical trials have not been performed.[26,50] In 1 report of 10 dogs treated with tacrolimus, 0.1% ointment applied to the perianal skin twice daily for 16 weeks, 5 dogs achieved complete resolution of lesions. Tacrolimus is more appropriate for topical application than cyclosporin A because of its smaller molecular weight, leading to improved absorption through the epidermis.[26] Because of the discomfort that may be associated with application, the author most commonly recommends topical tacrolimus ointment for dogs with mild lesions or for dogs with more severe lesions after complete or partial resolution with oral cyclosporin A (most often in combination with ketoconazole). Some dogs may be transitioned to topical tacrolimus ointment alone for maintenance to prevent relapses of perianal fistulas (**Fig. 4**).

Other Considerations for Medical Management

Dogs with active perianal fistulas can be painful, particularly on defecation.[2,3] Stool softeners should be considered, and, in some cases, enemas may be necessary to ease tenesmus. Analgesia should be prioritized for dogs with active lesions but the potential for constipation with use of some analgesics, such as opioid agonists,[53] should be considered when formulating a pain management plan. Some dogs with perianal fistulas are euthanized due to unremitting disease, development of complications such as anal stricture, or expense of long-term management.[43] For these reasons, early diagnosis and aggressive medical management of canine perianal fistulas are

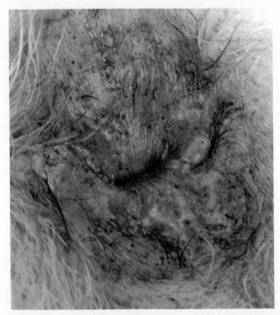

Fig. 4. Complete resolution of perianal sinus tracts in the 7-year-old German shepherd dog pictured in **Fig. 1**. This dog was treated with oral cyclosporin A and ketoconazole to the point of lesion resolution, then transitioned to topical tacrolimus 0.1% ointment. Clinical remission has been maintained for more than 12 months with application of tacrolimus ointment.

key. In the author's experience, management of patients with chronic lesions can be more challenging and these patients can be more refractory to medical therapy. Future studies should focus on better characterizing the genetics and immunopathogenesis of this disease, assessing quality of life of affected dogs and their owners (see Chiara Noli's article, "Assessing Quality of Life for Pets with Dermatologic Disease and their Owners," in this issue), and developing targeted medical therapies.

REFERENCES

1. Lee MJ, Parker CE, Taylor SR, et al. Efficacy of medical therapies for fistulizing Crohn's disease: a systematic review and meta-analysis. Clin Gastroenterol Hepatol 2018. https://doi.org/10.1016/j.cgh.2018.01.030.
2. Harkin KR, Walshaw R, Mullaney TP. Association of perianal fistula and colitis in the German shepherd dog: response to high-dose prednisone and dietary therapy. J Am Anim Hosp Assoc 1996;32:515–20.
3. Jamieson PM, Simpson JW, Kirby BM, et al. Association between anal furunculosis and colitis in the dog: preliminary observations. J Small Anim Pract 2002; 43:109–14.
4. Day MJ, Weaver BMQ. Pathology of surgically resected tissue from 305 cases of anal furunculosis in the dog. J Small Anim Pract 1992;33:583–9.
5. Killingsworth CR, Walshaw R, Dunstan RW, et al. Bacterial population and histologic changes in dogs with perianal fistula. Am J Vet Res 1988;49:1736–41.
6. House A, Gregory SP, Catchpole B. Expression of cytokine mRNA in canine anal furunculosis lesions. Vet Rec 2003;153:354–8.
7. House AK, Catchpole B, Gregory SP. Matrix metalloproteinase mRNA expression in canine anal furunculosis lesions. Vet Immunol Immunopathol 2007;115:68–75.
8. Tivers MS, Catchpole B, Gregory SP, et al. Interleukin-2 and interferon-gamma mRNA expression in canine anal furunculosis lesions and the effect of ciclosporin therapy. Vet Immunol Immunopathol 2008;125:31–6.
9. Lombardi RL, Marino DJ. Long-term evaluation of canine perianal fistula disease treated with exclusive fish and potato diet and surgical excision. J Am Anim Hosp Assoc 2008;44:302–7.
10. Ferrer L, Kimbrel EA, Lam A, et al. Treatment of perianal fistulas with human embryonic stem cell-derived mesenchymal stem cells: a canine model of human fistulizing Crohn's disease. Regen Med 2016;11:33–43.
11. Budsberg SC, Spurgeon TL, Liggitt HD. Anatomic predisposition to perianal fistulae formation in the German shepherd dog. Am J Vet Res 1985;46:1468–72.
12. Kennedy LJ, O'Neill T, House A, et al. Risk of anal furunculosis in German Shepherd dogs is associated with the major histocompatibility complex. Tissue Antigens 2007;71:51–6.
13. Olivry T, Rossi MA, Banovic F, et al. Mucocutaneous lupus erythematosus in dogs (21 cases). Vet Dermatol 2015;26:256-e55.
14. Scharl M, Rogler G, Bierdermann L. Fistulizing Crohn's disease. Clin Transl Gastroenterol 2017;8:e106.
15. Shelley BA. Use of the carbon dioxide laser for perianal and rectal surgery. Vet Clin Small Anim 2002;32:621–37.
16. Milner HR. The role of surgery in the management of canine anal furunculosis. A review of the literature and a retrospective evaluation of treatment by surgical resection in 51 dogs. N Z Vet J 2006;54:1–9.
17. Killingsworth CR, Walshaw R, Reimann KA, et al. Thyroid and immunologic status of dogs with perianal fistula. Am J Vet Res 1988;49:1742–6.

18. Day MJ. Immunopathology of anal furunculosis in the dog. J Small Anim Pract 1993;34:381–9.
19. Panés J, Rimola J. Perianal fistulizing Crohn's disease: pathogenesis, diagnosis and therapy. Nat Rev Gastroenterol Hepatol 2017;14:652–64.
20. House AK, Gregory SP, Catchpole B. Pattern-recognition receptor mRNA expression and function in canine monocyte/macrophages and relevance to canine anal furunculosis. Vet Immunol Immunopathol 2008;124:230–40.
21. Shearer DH, Day MJ. Aspects of the humoral immune response to Staphylococcus intermedius in dogs with superficial pyoderma, deep pyoderma and anal furunculosis. Vet Immunol Immunopathol 1997;58:107–20.
22. Vekic DA, Frew J, Cains GD. Hidradenitis suppurativa, a review of pathogenesis, associations and management. Part 1. Australas J Dermatol 2018. https://doi.org/10.1111/ajd.12770.
23. Lopetuso LR, Petito V, Zambrano D, et al. Gut microbiota: a key modulator of intestinal healing in inflammatory bowel disease. Dig Dis 2016;34:202–9.
24. Cammarota G, Pecere S, Ianiro G, et al. Principles of DNA-based gut microbiota assessment and therapeutic efficacy of fecal microbiota transplantation in gastrointestinal diseases. Dig Dis 2016;34:279–85.
25. Proverbio D, Perego R, Spada E, et al. Prevalence of adverse food reactions in 130 dogs in Italy with dermatologic signs: a retrospective study. J Small Anim Pract 2010;51:370–4.
26. Stanley BJ, Hauptman JG. Long-term prospective evaluation of topically applied 0.1% tacrolimus ointment for treatment of perianal sinuses in dogs. J Am Vet Med Assoc 2009;235:397–404.
27. Barnes A, O'Neill T, Kennedy LJ, et al. Association of canine anal furunculosis with TNFA is secondary to linkage disequilibrium with DLA-DRB1. Tissue Antigens 2009;73:218–24.
28. Massey J, Short AD, Catchpole B, et al. Genetics of canine anal furunculosis in the German shepherd dog. Immunogenetics 2014;66:311–24.
29. House AK, Binns MM, Gregory SP, et al. Analysis of NOD1, NOD2, TLR1, TLR2, TLR4, TLR5, TLR6 and TLR9 genes in anal furunculosis of German shepherd dogs. Tissue Antigens 2009;73:250–4.
30. Vekic DA, Cains GD. Hidradenitis suppurativa, a review of pathogenesis, associations and management. Part 2. Australas J Dermatol 2018. https://doi.org/10.1111/ajd.12766.
31. Lukach AJ, Saul MI, Ferris LK, et al. Risk factors for hidradenitis suppurativa in patients with inflammatory bowel disease. Dig Dis Sci 2018;63:755–60.
32. Adegbola SO, Pisani A, Sahnan K, et al. Medical and surgical management of perianal Crohn's disease. Ann Gastroenterol 2018;31:129–39.
33. Schlapbach C, Hanni T, Yalwalkar N, et al. Expression of the IL-23/Th17 pathway in lesions of hidradenitis suppurativa. J Am Acad Dermatol 2011;65:790–8.
34. Vasseur PB. Results of surgical excision of perianal fistulas in dogs. J Am Vet Med Assoc 1984;185:60–2.
35. Klein A, Deneuche A, Fayolle P, et al. Preoperative immunosuppressive therapy and surgery as a treatment for anal furunculosis. Vet Surg 2006;25:759–68.
36. Ellison GW, Bellah JR, Stubbs WP, et al. Treatment of perianal fistulas with ND:YAG laser – results in twenty cases. Vet Surg 1995;24:140–7.
37. Budsberg SC, Robinette JD, Farrell RK. Cryotherapy performed on perianal fistulas in dogs (Washington State University 1976-1980). Vet Med Small Anim Clin 1981;76:667–9.

38. Tisdall PLC, Hunt GB, Beck JA, et al. Management of perianal fistulae in five dogs using azathioprine and metronidazole prior to surgery. Aust Vet J 1999;77:374–8.
39. Becker E, Bengs S, Aluri S, et al. Doxycycline, metronidazole and isotretinoin: do they modify microRNA/mRNA expression profiles and function in murine T-cells? Sci Rep 2016;6:37082.
40. Harkin KR, Phillips D, Wilkerson M. Evaluation of azathioprine on lesion severity and lymphocyte blastogenesis in dogs with perianal fistulas. J Am Anim Hosp Assoc 2007;43:21–6.
41. Mathews KA, Sukhiani HR. Randomized controlled trial of cyclosporine for treatment of perianal fistulas in dogs. J Am Vet Med Assoc 1997;211:1249–53.
42. Mathews KA, Ayres SA, Tano CA, et al. Cyclosporin treatment of perianal fistulas in dogs. Can Vet J 1997;38:39–41.
43. Griffiths LG, Sullivan M, Borland WW. Cyclosporin as the sole treatment for anal furunculosis: preliminary results. J Small Anim Pract 1999;40:569–72.
44. House AK, Guitian J, Gregory SP, et al. Evaluation of the effect of two dose rates of cyclosporine on the severity of perianal fistulae lesions and associated clinical signs in dogs. Vet Surg 2006;35:543–9.
45. Hardie RJ, Gregory SP, Tomlin J, et al. Cyclosporine treatment of anal furunculosis in 26 dogs. J Small Anim Pract 2005;46:3–9.
46. Doust R, Griffiths LG, Sullivan M. Evaluation of once daily treatment with cyclosporine for anal furunculosis in dogs. Vet Rec 2003;152:225–9.
47. Patricelli AJ, Hardie RJ, McAnulty JF. Cyclosporine and ketoconazole for the treatment of perianal fistulas in dogs. J Am Vet Med Assoc 2002;220:1009–16.
48. Mouatt JG. Cyclosporin and ketoconazole interaction for treatment of perianal fistulas in the dog. Aust Vet J 2002;80:207–11.
49. O'Neill T, Edwards GA, Holloway S. Efficacy of combined cyclosporine A and ketoconazole for treatment of anal furunculosis. J Small Anim Pract 2004;45:238–43.
50. Misseghers BS, Binnington AG, Mathews KA. Clinical observations of the treatment of canine perianal fistulas with topical tacrolimus in 10 dogs. Can Vet J 2000;41:623–7.
51. Ackermann AL, May ER, Frank LA. Use of mycophenolate mofetil to treat immune-mediated skin disease in 14 dogs – a retrospective evaluation. Vet Dermatol 2017;195-e44.
52. Palmeiro BS. Cyclosporine in veterinary dermatology. Vet Clin North Am Small Anim Pract 2013;43:153–71.
53. Epstein M, Rodan I, Griffenhagen G, et al. 2015 AAHA/AAFP pain management guidelines for dogs and cats. J Am Anim Hosp Assoc 2015;51:67–84.

Canine and Feline Cutaneous Epitheliotropic Lymphoma and Cutaneous Lymphocytosis

Kathryn A. Rook, VMD

KEYWORDS

- Cutaneous epitheliotropic lymphoma • Cutaneous T-cell lymphoma
- Cutaneous lymphocytosis • T lymphocyte • Mycosis fungoides • Sézary syndrome
- Pagetoid reticulosis

KEY POINTS

- Canine epitheliotropic T-cell lymphoma is an uncommon neoplastic disease with a poor prognosis and poor response to treatment.
- Feline epitheliotropic lymphoma is a rare neoplastic disease believed to carry a poor prognosis.
- Cutaneous lymphocytosis is considered a rare, indolent disease in dogs and cats with potential for transformation to malignant lymphoma.

CANINE CUTANEOUS EPITHELIOTROPIC LYMPHOMA
Clinical Presentation

Canine cutaneous epitheliotropic lymphoma, also known as cutaneous T-cell lymphoma (CTCL), is an uncommon and often fatal neoplastic condition.[1–3] This disease typically affects older dogs with no sex predilection and is said to represent less than 1% of all skin tumors.[3] Currently, this disease has an unknown cause.[1] Many published studies also show no breed predisposition.[4,5] However, several older studies have indicated that English cocker spaniels and boxers may be predisposed.[6–10] One recent case series had an overrepresentation of golden retriever dogs.[11] The clinical and histopathologic features described in the human form of this disease are applied generally to its canine counterparts to divide it into three subforms: (1) mycosis fungoides (MF), named for the mushroom-like appearance of the skin tumors; (2) pagetoid reticulosis (PR); and (3) Sézary syndrome.[2]

Clinically, dogs with MF have varying lesion types including generalized exfoliative erythroderma (characterized by generalized erythema, scaling, and pruritus),

Disclosure Statement: The author has nothing to disclose.
Department of Clinical Sciences and Advanced Medicine, School of Veterinary Medicine, University of Pennsylvania, 3900 Delancey Street, Philadelphia, PA 19104, USA
E-mail address: karook@vet.upenn.edu

Vet Clin Small Anim 49 (2019) 67–81
https://doi.org/10.1016/j.cvsm.2018.08.007
0195-5616/19/© 2018 Elsevier Inc. All rights reserved.

mucocutaneous lesions with depigmentation, erosions or ulcers, solitary or multiple cutaneous nodules or plaques throughout the skin, or infiltrative oral mucosal disease (**Figs. 1** and **2**).[1,2] More recently a case report has also indicated that vesiculobullous lesions are seen with epitheliotropic lymphoma in dogs.[12] Humans with MF tend to progress from the patch or plaque stage to more generalized exfoliative erythroderma and/or development of tumors, whereas in canine patients with MF, the variety of lesions can present at any time during disease development and each lesion type does not represent a progressive disease stage.[13,14]

Sézary syndrome is a progressive form of MF during which patients become leukemic and neoplastic lymphocytes are found in the peripheral blood. These neoplastic lymphocytes are called Sézary cells and have a characteristic appearance with cerebriform nuclei. Sézary syndrome is thought to be extremely rare in dogs,[7,15] but represents approximately 5% of cases of human CTCLs.[16]

Dogs with PR present with similar clinical signs as those with MF.[17] The difference in subtype is based solely on histopathology. Histopathologically, dogs with PR have a neoplastic infiltrate present solely within the epidermis and adnexal structures, whereas those with MF have neoplastic cells also present within the underlying dermis.[2] There are two forms of PR, a localized form, also called the Woringer-Kolopp form, and a generalized form, known as the Ketron-Goodman form.[13]

Although patients with CTCL presenting with a combination of lesions are usually not a diagnostic challenge, patients with small areas of erythroderma or with a few

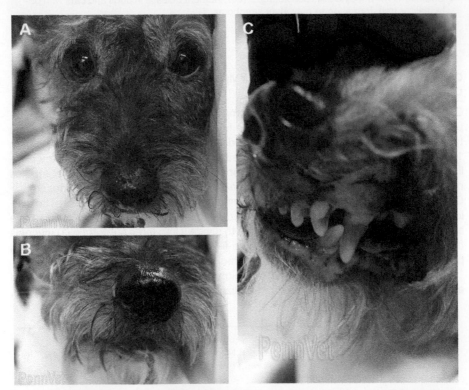

Fig. 1. Clinical signs associated with epitheliotropic cutaneous lymphoma. (*A*) Depigmentation of the periocular mucosae. (*B*) Depigmentation of the nasal planum and alar folds. (*C*) Depigmentation of the lip margins.

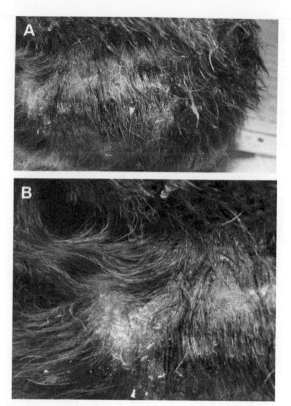

Fig. 2. (*A, B*) Exfoliative erythroderma.

plaques or patches are often presumed to be presenting with allergic dermatitis.[18] Most dogs with CTCL are also pruritic, which may lead to the inclusion of differential diagnoses, such as ectoparasitic infestations, allergic dermatitis, or secondary skin infections.[1,18] Obtaining a thorough and complete history often reveals no prior history of allergic skin disease in these older patients or only minor signs of pruritus in the past.[18] Additionally, a careful physical examination may reveal less obvious lesions that are more suggestive of CTCL, such as mild depigmentation of mucous membranes and footpads.[1] One study has indicated a potential connection between allergic dermatitis and development of cutaneous lymphoma; however, a true association has not been proven (**Table 1**).[19]

Diagnosis

In cases where ulcerated plaques or nodules are present, performing skin surface cytology is often the initial recommended step.[17] This helps to find evidence of secondary bacterial skin infections, which are not uncommon in cases of CTCL. In some cases, lymphocytes may be evident on surface cytology; however, skin biopsy is still necessary in most cases to reach a diagnosis.[17]

The definitive diagnosis of CTCL can only be made by dermatohistopathology.[1,2,17] To diagnose epitheliotropic lymphoma, neoplastic T cells must demonstrate tropism for the epidermal or mucosal epithelium and adnexal structures. Neoplastic lymphocytes are evenly distributed throughout the epidermis, but may also be found within

Table 1
Comparison of disease characteristics

	Clinical Presentation	Histopathology	Phenotype	Prognosis	Recommended Therapies
Canine epitheliotropic cutaneous lymphoma	Exfoliative erythroderma Patches/plaques Tumors Depigmentation of mucocutaneous junctions Most often pruritic	Medium-to-large lymphocytes within all layers of epidermis Neoplastic lymphocytes often invade adnexae Pautrier's microabscesses	Most often CD8$^+$ T cells Most often gamma/delta T cells	Poor Median 6-mo survival time	Hollywood brand safflower oil Isotretinoin or etretinate More studies necessary to determine efficacy of lomustine, bexarotene, histone deacetylase inhibitors, and rabacofosadine
Feline epitheliotropic cutaneous lymphoma	Exfoliative erythroderma Patches/plaques Variable pruritus	Neoplastic lymphocytes vary from small to large Variable infiltration of adnexae Pautrier's microabscesses can be present	Unknown Believed to be of cytotoxic T-cell origin	Poor Median survival time reported as 10.25 mo	Unknown efficacy of any chemotherapeutic agents on survival time
Cutaneous lymphocytosis	Cats: erythematous scaly plaques, nodules, or papules over the thorax; often focal lesion Dogs: erythema with alopecia and scaling; often multifocal lesions	Lymphocytic infiltrate within superficial dermis Dogs: grenz zone present Cats: 50% have infiltration of epidermis and adnexae	T cells 50% of cases contain small aggregates of B cells within lymphocytic infiltrate	Variable May progress to malignant lymphoma	Glucocorticoids?

small, discrete aggregates known as Pautrier's microabscesses or microaggregates with in the upper layers of the epidermis (**Fig. 3**). In patch and plaque stage lesions, neoplastic lymphocytes may be small-to-medium sized and can resemble mature lymphocytes, whereas in the tumor stage, infiltrating cells are usually intermediate to large.[2] Unfortunately, in some early cases, the neoplastic infiltrate may resemble the inflammation seen with an interface dermatitis, such as erythema multiforme. In these cases, repeating skin biopsies as the disease progresses clinically often allows for and may be necessary for a more definitive diagnosis.[2,7,20] However, this diagnostic dilemma has successfully led some individuals to create primers for polymerase chain reaction to identify clonality of lymphocytic infiltrates in these difficult to diagnose cases.[21]

Immunohistochemistry and Immunopathology

Although much of clinical and histopathologic descriptions regarding canine CTCL are adapted from the human form of the disease, canine and human MF exhibit marked differences in T-cell subtypes among the malignant population. It is known that 90% of human CTCLs have T cells bearing the CD4 cell surface marker, whereas 80% to 90% of canine patients possess the CD8 marker, and the remainder are generally CD4 negative and CD8 negative.[10,22] These two cell surface markers are often used to differentiate between T-cell subtypes: CD4+ T cells are classically believed to be the part of the T helper (Th) subtype, whereas CD8+ T cells are usually of the cytotoxic subtype.[23] Additionally, most T cells from human patients with CTCL bear the alpha/beta T-cell receptor, whereas canine neoplastic cells carry the gamma/delta T-cell receptor in approximately 62% of cases.[10] Infrequently, humans with CTCL have neoplastic T cells with the cell surface markers that are more typical of canine disease (CD8+ and/or gamma/delta T-cell receptors). Humans with gamma/delta or aggressive cytotoxic phenotypes have an especially poor prognosis.[24–27] Similarly, canine cutaneous lymphoma carries a poor prognosis (discussed later).[1–3]

The neoplastic lymphocytes in human MF are most commonly CD4+ with the alpha/beta T-cell receptor. In addition, it is well known that these neoplastic cells are skewed toward a Th2-type cytokine phenotype in Sézary syndrome.[14,28] Studies have shown increases in interleukin (IL)-4 and IL-13 production in stimulated circulating Sézary

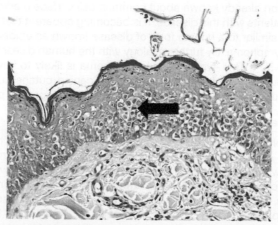

Fig. 3. Histopathology of epitheliotropic lymphoma in a dog. Neoplastic lymphocytes infiltrate all layers of the epidermis. Arrow shows Pautrier's microabscess. (H&E, 10× magnification). (*Courtesy of* Dr. Michael Goldschmidt, Hilton Head, SC.)

cells and increases in mRNA production of IL-4 and IL-5 in clinically affected skin.[14] However, levels of IL-12 and interferon (IFN)-α in the peripheral blood manifested a progressive decline, which correlated with decreases in the numbers and functions of circulating dendritic cells.[14] However, understanding this immunologic imbalance has allowed for various successful therapeutic approaches, including the direct administration of IFN-α or -γ or IL-12, which can lead to amelioration of the immunologic milieu.[29–33]

More recently, a study evaluated the presence of CD25+ T cells in various subtypes of canine lymphomas and the potential relationship with prognosis.[34] Although samples from only two patients with CTCL were obtained, they both showed increased presence of CD25+ T cells within the lymphocytic infiltrates.[34] CD25 is also known as the IL-2 receptor alpha chain, which is one component of a three subunit IL-2 receptor present on the surface of T cells. The presence of the IL-2 receptor on the T-cell surface allows for high-affinity binding of IL-2, which leads to proliferation and maturation of lymphocytes.[35] In humans with CTCL, high rates of CD25+ T cells have also been reported[36,37] and this has correlated with metastasis and histologic grade.[36] The results of the canine study may also be indicative that the presence of CD25 may be associated with a poor prognosis.[34]

Other than the few cell markers that have been investigated, the immunophenotype of canine cutaneous lymphoma has not yet been fully elucidated. Recently, a small study was published evaluating upregulation of cytokine and chemokine mRNA in the skin of seven patients diagnosed with cutaneous epitheliotropic lymphoma. Although the number of patients was small, the transcription levels of the Th-1 type cytokines IL-12 and IFN-γ were increased in affected skin as compared with normal skin.[38] Additionally, levels of cytotoxic T-cell markers, perforin and granzyme B, which are typically associated with CD8+ cytotoxic T cells, were higher in lesional skin as compared with normal skin.[38] The author has also performed a small pilot study showing increased mRNA production of IFN-γ and tumor necrosis factor-α in affected skin of a small number of patients with cutaneous lymphoma (Kathryn A. Rook, VMD, unpublished data). Additional studies still must be performed with larger patient populations and with assays that equate increased gene transcription to protein production to further understand the immunopathogenesis of CTCL in dogs.

Based on the small studies performed by the author and Chimura and colleagues[38] and the information already known about common cell surface markers in neoplastic cells in canine patients with this disease, it is becoming apparent that the canine form of CTCL is most similar to a human form of disease known as epidermotropic CD8+ cytotoxic T-cell lymphoma. By further analogy with the human disease, administering IFN to patients with a Th-1-type cytotoxic lymphoma is likely to have a detrimental effect. Further elucidation of the pathogenesis of canine cutaneous epitheliotropic lymphoma may allow for more targeted therapies and an improved prognosis.

Prognosis and Treatment

The prognosis for patients with epitheliotropic lymphoma is poor. The reported survival times after diagnosis with CTCL are anywhere from a few months to up to 2 years.[6,39] However, the median survival time in one study was reported as 6 months.[18] A more recent retrospective study of 148 dogs found an overall survival time of 264 days. Dogs in this study with only cutaneous lesions had a survival time of 130 days compared with 491 days for those patients with mucosal lesions.[11] Unfortunately, despite treatment of this disease, the overall survival time may not be significantly altered.[17] Death caused by dissemination of the disease is rare, but can occur.[40] Most clients request humane euthanasia because of poor quality of life, which is often related to development of many ulcerated skin tumors, severe secondary skin infections, and/or marked unmanageable pruritus.[17] This is in stark contrast to human MF, where the prognosis is good; those patients without Sézary syndrome have an estimated survival rate after 5 years of 89% to 93% with treatment.[41,42] The prognosis for dogs with this disease is, however, similar to the prognosis for human patients with epidermotropic $CD8^+$ cytotoxic T-cell lymphoma. Those human patients have a median 5-year survival rate of only 32%.[43]

Several different treatment protocols have been suggested for dogs with CTCL, including many that revolve around the commonly used CHOP-based protocols for treatment of lymphoma and other common chemotherapeutic agents. These may allow for improved quality of life for some time, but often do not improve survival times.[17] However, in the 2017 retrospective study by Chan and colleagues,[11] dogs with cutaneous lesions receiving chemotherapeutic interventions did have a longer median survival time compared with those not receiving therapy. One retrospective study evaluated response of CTCL in 46 dogs to treatment with lomustine, an alkylating agent. In this study, 14 dogs received lomustine as their sole therapy, whereas greater than half (27 of 43 dogs) received treatment with glucocorticoids concurrently, and five dogs also received at least one dose of L-asparaginase. The starting treatment dose of lomustine was 60 mg/m^2 and ranged from 30 to 95 mg/m^2. Fifteen dogs achieved a complete remission, 23 had a partial remission, five had stable disease, and three had progressive disease. The response duration was 94 days with a range of 22 to 282 days.[4] Based on this study, lomustine is a common first agent for treatment, although this recommendation has become controversial in the recent past.[44] Given that this recommendation has been made based on reports of response in small numbers of dogs and retrospective studies, additional prospective studies with a larger patient population are recommended.

Other treatment options recommended based on small patient numbers include safflower oil, oral retinoids, pegylated doxorubicin, rabacfosadine, and total skin electron beam therapy.[45–50] Six of eight dogs that received 3 mL/kg of Hollywood foods brand safflower achieved remission with minimal side effects and no concurrent therapies.[45] Similarly, a small number of dogs achieved remission after receiving either oral isotretinoin or etretinate, both systemic retinoids.[46] In the recent retrospective study evaluating clinical outcomes, patients with multiple cutaneous lesions receiving retinoids had a longer median survival time compared with those that did not receive retinoids.[11] It is noteworthy that the neoplastic cells in canine CTCL do possess both types of retinoid receptors (RAR, RXR), indicating that these may be potential targets for improved therapies.[51] In fact, use of bexarotene, a newer generation retinoid that activates the RXR receptor, and which is highly effective for human CTCL, is a drug that may be beneficial for treatment of canine patients.[52] No formal studies evaluating efficacy in canine patients have been performed to date, likely because of the high cost of the drug.

Pegylated doxorubicin is a liposomal encapsulated form of the antineoplastic antibiotic doxorubicin. This form of doxorubicin was evaluated in patients with various neoplastic diseases, including nine with cutaneous lymphoma. Out of these nine patients, three had a complete response and one had a partial response to treatment,[1] again indicating that additional efficacy studies need to be performed with larger patient populations. Pegylated doxorubicin was evaluated because of decreased risk of cardiac toxicity and greater cytotoxicity for some neoplastic cell types.[47]

A new drug, called rabacfosadine, previously known as VDC-1101 and GS-9219, has recently been conditionally approved by the Food and Drug Administration in the United States for treatment of lymphoma in dogs. This medication is part of the acyclic nucleoside phosphonates, which are often recognized as antiviral medications used for the treatment of human immunodeficiency virus. Rabacfosadine is a propro-drug of [9-(2-phosphonylmethoxyethyl)guanine] (PMEG). It is phosphorylated twice to its active metabolite PMEGpp. This active metabolite has cytotoxic activity by acting on and inhibiting DNA polymerases and by incorporating PMEG into DNA.[49] One clin-ical trial has been performed in 12 patients with cutaneous lymphoma that received rabacfosadine in combination with prednisone at 1 mg/kg every other day. Ten of 12 patients receiving this medication had CTCL, whereas the others were diagnosed with nonepitheliotropic cutaneous lymphoma. The objective response rate (the per-centage of dogs with either a complete remission or a partial remission) was 45%. When including those patients with stable disease, the biologic response rate was 64%. Although the one dog in this study that experienced a complete remission was diagnosed with nonepitheliotropic lymphoma, this new drug may offer another treatment option to improve the quality of life of those patients with CTCL.[48]

Finally, a recent case report indicated that total skin electron beam therapy was use-ful for palliative therapy in one patient. This therapy has been well-documented as an effective treatment option for humans with MF and again should be more formally evaluated for canine patients with this disease.[50]

Several other therapies are available for humans with CD8+ epidermotropic cyto-toxic T-cell lymphoma including histone deacetylase (HDAC) inhibitors and allogenic bone marrow transplantation.[53] HDAC inhibitors inhibit tumor growth by modulating and inhibiting gene transcription. Vorinostat and romidepsin, both HDAC inhibitors, have been approved for treatment of humans with cutaneous lymphoma. In vitro studies on effects of HDAC inhibitors on canine cancer lines have shown promise in the treatment of lymphoma.[54] Pharmacokinetic and pharmacodynamics studies have been performed in dogs for some HDAC inhibitors; however, clinical trials for evaluation of efficacy in epitheliotropic lymphoma are few in number.[55] It is likely that, although these therapies may be useful, they are currently cost prohibitive in vet-erinary medicine.

FELINE EPITHELTIOTROPIC CUTANEOUS T-CELL LYMPHOMA

Although some information is available regarding cutaneous lymphoma in dogs, far less is available regarding this disease in feline patients. Similar to dogs, epithelio-tropic and nonepitheliotropic forms of the disease exist, again characterized by the location of neoplastic lymphocytes on histopathology.[1,2] This section focuses on epi-theliotropic cutaneous lymphoma in cats.

Clinical Presentation

Epitheliotropic cutaneous lymphoma is an extremely rare neoplasm in the cat. To date, few cases have been reported in the literature.[56] The median age of onset is approx-imately 13.5 years with no apparent breed or sex predilection.[56] Clinically, cats with this disease can present with signs similar to those in dogs including exfoliative eryth-roderma, patches, plaques, erosions, ulcers, and lesions in the oral cavity and at mucocutaneous junctions (**Fig. 4**).[2,56] According to older reports, lesions most often affected the face, eyelids, mucocutaneous junctions, elbows, and trunk.[2] A more recent update to the literature including new cases indicated that single or multifocal lesions could be present with no predilection for a particular body site.[56] As in dogs, clinical signs can resemble those of other diseases including allergic skin disease manifesting as part of the eosinophilic granuloma complex, such as eosinophilic plaques.[56]

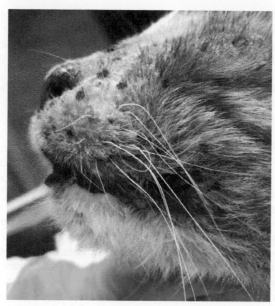

Fig. 4. Alopecia, erythema, scaling, and a focal ulcer in a cat with epitheliotropic cutaneous lymphoma.

In contrast to dogs with cutaneous lymphoma, the presence of pruritus is variable in cats and the disease is usually slowly progressive.[56] Sézary syndrome, or the leukemic variant of epitheliotropic lymphoma, has been reported in two cats.[57,58] Additionally, cats diagnosed with cutaneous epitheliotropic lymphoma are rarely positive for feline leukemia virus infection.[59–61]

Diagnosis

Definitive diagnosis of epitheliotropic cutaneous lymphoma in cats is also made via dermatohistopathology. Small-to-medium or medium-to-large neoplastic lymphocytes with tropism for the epidermis must be seen to make the diagnosis.[2] In some cases, neoplastic lymphocytes also invade the adnexae[2]; however, in the five most recently reported cases in the literature, this was not a feature on histopathology.[56] Pautrier's microabscesses are a histopathologic feature, but are not found in every reported case of feline epitheliotropic lymphoma.[56]

Immunohistochemistry and Immunopathology

Unfortunately, little is known about the immunophenotype and immunopathology in feline cutaneous epitheliotropic cutaneous lymphoma. Immunostaining for CD4 and CD8 to differentiate between T-helper subtypes has historically not been possible on formalin-fixed, paraffin-embedded feline tissue. Some pathologists speculate that the immunophenotype of feline disease is most similar to human MF rather than canine CTCL in that it is more likely to be CD4[+] rather than CD8[+].[56] However, Neta and colleagues[62] reported on one case of feline epitheliotropic cutaneous lymphoma that had positive cytoplasmic staining for perforin. Perforin is a protein stored within cytoplasmic granules of cytotoxic T lymphocytes and natural killer cells along with granzymes. Perforin is responsible for forming pores in cell membranes and granzymes then flow through these channels to perform targeted killing of cells by cytotoxic T lymphocytes and natural killer cells.[23] In this published case report, neoplastic cells also stained positively for CD3 indicating they were of T-cell origin. Again, because of the lack of freshly frozen tissue, additional immunostaining for CD4 and CD8 could not be performed in this individual patient.[62]

As in dogs, it is hoped that further characterization of the immunophenotype of feline disease will allow for better understanding of the pathogenesis of disease and for developing more targeted therapies.

Prognosis and Treatment

The prognosis for feline epitheliotropic lymphoma is also believed to be poor. The median survival time for six patients diagnosed with this disease was reported in the literature as 10.25 months with a range of 2.5 months to 4 years.[57,58,62–64] In the more recent case series of 15 feline patients, the survival time was not determined, but was estimated to be only between 1 and 6 months, making it similar to what is seen in canine patients.[56]

Likely because of the small number of reported cases and rarity of the disease in cats, no clinical trials or retrospective analyses of treatment options have been performed. Some recommend the same dose of lomustine that is used in dogs should also be used for treatment of cats with epitheliotropic lymphoma.[4,5,62] However, several other treatments have been attempted including surgery; electron-beam irradiation; a combination of vincristine and cyclophosphamide; and either intravenous or intralesional injections of fibronectin, which is a high-molecular-weight glycoprotein that is part of the extracellular matrix and has been reported to have effects on neoplastic cells.[57,63] These treatment options have had varying efficacy. Additional studies are recommended to determine which type of therapy is most effective in treatment of feline epitheliotropic lymphoma.

CANINE AND FELINE CUTANEOUS LYMPHOCYTOSIS

In human medicine, the term cutaneous pseudolymphoma is used to describe various benign skin conditions that either clinically or histopathologically resemble lymphomas. Other terms used to describe this disease include lymphocytoma cutis and cutaneous lymphoid hyperplasia, which has become the preferred terminology. In the case of humans, this disease is most often idiopathic in nature, but associations have been made with various antigen exposures, such as insect bites, bacterial or viral infections, tattoos, vaccines, or medications. Clinically, humans with cutaneous lymphoid hyperplasia most often present with a single or localized area of violaceous papules, plaques, or nodules. Histopathologically, there is a nodular to diffuse dermal infiltrate of lymphocytes with the epidermis being separated from the dermis by a grenz zone, a narrow area of unaffected dermis. The lymphoid population can either be a mix of B and T lymphocytes or mostly T lymphocytes. In many cases there is spontaneous regression of disease or slow progression of disease without metastasis; however, occasionally progression to lymphoma can occur.[13]

In veterinary medicine, cutaneous lymphocytosis (CL) has been adopted to describe this particular rare disease process.[2,65] Unlike cutaneous epitheliotropic lymphoma, CL has been reported more commonly in the cat than the dog.[2] On average, cats become affected between 12 and 13 years of age.[1,2,65,66] There is no breed predilection; however, female cats may be slightly more predisposed to developing this disease.[65] Only a small number of cases have been reported in dogs. Similar to cats this was seen in an older population of dogs, approximately 8 years old. Because of the small number of reported cases, no breed or sex predilections are made in the dog.[67]

Cats most often present with a single lesion of erythema with scale and alopecia with or without crusting.[65,66] Occasionally, erythematous and scaly plaques, nodules, or papules are seen. Lesions are most common over the thorax, but are seen anywhere on the body, with the legs, pinnae, flank, and neck being other common locations. Cats with CL are often pruritic.[65] Dogs with CL are reported to present with multifocal lesions of erythema with alopecia, scaling, and occasionally plaques. Although nodules and papules have been reported in cats and humans, this is not a feature that has been seen in dogs with CL. Similarly, pruritus is rarely a feature of disease in dogs.[67]

Diagnosis of CL in dogs and cats is by histopathology. A lymphocytic infiltrate is present predominantly in the superficial dermis and in dogs, as in humans, a grenz zone is present and often spares the adnexae and epithelium.[2] In cats, there is intraepidermal and intrafollicular lymphocytes in about half of cases.[65] The dermal infiltrate in dogs and cats is comprised mainly of small lymphocytes with rare to absent mitotic figures.[2] In feline disease, most lymphocytes within the infiltrate are T cells, expressing CD18, CD3, and CD5.[65] In about half of cases in cats and dogs there are small aggregates of B cells within the lymphocytic infiltrate.[65,67]

Immunohistochemistry has been performed on five canine samples. Results indicate that, unlike with CTCL, T-cell receptors of the alpha/beta subtype are more common in CL. About half coexpressed CD8 or lacked CD4 and CD8.[67]

Various treatments have been attempted with different outcomes. In dogs and cats, treatment with glucocorticoids has been most common.[65–67] It has previously been reported that 14 of 18 cats treated with systemic or topical glucocorticoids showed some response to therapy. With failure of glucocorticoids, chlorambucil or lomustine have been used, again with four of five cats responding.[1,65] Despite varying response to therapy in dogs and cats, CL is most often considered an indolent disease; however, transformation to malignant lymphoma can occur in both species with time. In these cases, prognosis is generally poor.[65,67]

REFERENCES

1. Miller WH, Griffin CE, Campbell KL, et al. Muller & Kirk's small animal dermatology. 7th edition. St. Louis (MO): Elsevier; 2013. p. 938.
2. Gross TL, Gross TL. Skin diseases of the dog and cat: clinical and histopathologic diagnosis. Ames (IA): Blackwell Science; 2005. p. 932.
3. Cutaneous lymphosarcoma. In: Goldschmidt MH, Shofer FS, editors. Skin tumors of the dog and cat. 1st edition. Boston: Reed Educational and Professional Publishing Ltd; 1998. p. 252–64.
4. Risbon RE, Lorimier LP, Skorupski K, et al. Response of canine cutaneous epitheliotropic lymphoma to lomustine (CCNU): a retrospective study of 46 cases (1999–2004). J Vet Intern Med 2006;20(6):1389–97.
5. Williams LE, Rassnick KM, Power HT, et al. CCNU in the treatment of canine epitheliotropic lymphoma. J Vet Intern Med 2006;20(1):136–43.
6. Beale KM, Bolon B. Canine cutaneous lymphosarcoma epitheliotropic and non epitheliotropic, a retrospective study. In: Ihrke PJ, Mason IS, White SD, editors. Advances in veterinary dermatology. New York: Pergamon Press; 1993. p. 273–84.
7. Foster AP, Evans E, Kerlin RL, et al. Cutaneous T-cell lymphoma with Sézary syndrome in a dog. Vet Clin Pathol 1997;26(4):188–92.

8. Bhang DH, Choi US, Kim MK, et al. Epitheliotropic cutaneous lymphoma (mycosis fungoides) in a dog. J Vet Sci 2006;7(1):97–9.
9. Day MJ. Immunophenotypic characterization of cutaneous lymphoid neoplasia in the dog and cat. J Comp Pathol 1995;112(1):79–96.
10. Moore PF, Olivry T, Naydan D. Canine cutaneous epitheliotropic lymphoma (mycosis fungoides) is a proliferative disorder of CD8+ T cells. Am J Pathol 1994;144(2):421–9.
11. Chan CM, Frimberger AE, Moore AS. Clinical outcome and prognosis of dogs with histopathological features consistent with epitheliotropic lymphoma: a retrospective study of 148 cases (2003-2015). Vet Dermatol 2018;29(2):e59.
12. Bizikova P, Linder KE, Suter SE, et al. Canine cutaneous epitheliotropic T-cell lymphoma with vesiculobullous lesions resembling human bullous mycosis fungoides. Vet Dermatol 2009;20(4):281–8.
13. Fitzpatrick TB, Wolff K. Fitzpatrick's dermatology in general medicine. 7th edition. New York: McGraw-Hill Medical; 2008. p. 136.
14. Kim EJ, Lin J, Junkins-Hopkins JM, et al. Mycosis fungoides and Sezary syndrome: an update. Curr Oncol Rep 2006;8(5):376–86.
15. Moore PF, Olivry T. Cutaneous lymphomas in companion animals. Clin Dermatol 1994;12(4):499–505.
16. Hwang ST, Janik JE, Jaffe ES, et al. Mycosis fungoides and Sezary syndrome. Lancet 2008;371(9616):945–57.
17. Fontaine J, Bovens C, Bettenay S, et al. Canine cutaneous epitheliotropic T-cell lymphoma: a review. Vet Comp Oncol 2009;7(1):1–14.
18. Fontaine J, Heimann M, Day MJ. Canine cutaneous epitheliotropic T-cell lymphoma: a review of 30 cases. Vet Dermatol 2010;21(3):267–75.
19. Santoro D, Marsella R, Hernandez J. Investigation on the association between atopic dermatitis and the development of mycosis fungoides in dogs: a retrospective case-control study. Vet Dermatol 2007;18(2):101–6.
20. Murphy MK, Thierry O. Comparison of T-lymphocyte proliferation in canine epitheliotropic lymphosarcoma and benign lymphocytic dermatoses. Vet Dermatol 2000;11(2):99–105.
21. Chaubert P, Baur Chaubert AS, Sattler U, et al. Improved polymerase chain reaction-based method to detect early-stage epitheliotropic T-cell lymphoma (mycosis fungoides) in formalin-fixed, paraffin-embedded skin biopsy specimens of the dog. J Vet Diagn Invest 2010;22(1):20–9.
22. Knowles DM. Immunophenotypic and antigen receptor gene rearrangement analysis in T cell neoplasia. Am J Pathol 1989;134(4):761–86.
23. Abbas AK, Lichtman AH, Pillai S, et al. Cellular and molecular immunology. 9th edition. Philadelphia: Elsevier; 2018.
24. Diwan H, Ivan D. CD8-positive mycosis fungoides and primary cutaneous aggressive epidermotropic CD8-positive cytotoxic T-cell lymphoma. J Cutan Pathol 2009;36(3):390–2.
25. Berti E, Tomasini D, Vermeer MH, et al. Primary cutaneous CD8-positive epidermotropic cytotoxic T cell lymphomas. A distinct clinicopathological entity with an aggressive clinical behavior. Am J Pathol 1999;155(2):483–92.
26. Toro JR, Beaty M, Sorbara L, et al. Gamma delta T-cell lymphoma of the skin: a clinical, microscopic, and molecular study. Arch Dermatol 2000;136(8):1024–32.
27. Lu D, Patel KA, Duvic M, et al. Clinical and pathological spectrum of CD8-positive cutaneous T-cell lymphomas. J Cutan Pathol 2002;29(8):465–72.

28. Vowels BR, Lessin SR, Cassin M, et al. Th2 cytokine mRNA expression in skin in cutaneous T-cell lymphoma. J Invest Dermatol 1994;103(5):669–73.
29. Rook AH, Wood GS, Yoo EK, et al. Interleukin-12 therapy of cutaneous T-cell lymphoma induces lesion regression and cytotoxic T-cell responses. Blood 1999; 94(3):902–8.
30. Rook AH, Gottlieb SL, Wolfe JT, et al. Pathogenesis of cutaneous T-cell lymphoma: implications for the use of recombinant cytokines and photopheresis. Clin Exp Immunol 1997;107(Suppl 1):16–20.
31. Rook AH, Kuzel TM, Olsen EA. Cytokine therapy of cutaneous T-cell lymphoma: interferons, interleukin-12, and interleukin-2. Hematol Oncol Clin North Am 2003; 17(6):48, ix.
32. Rook AH, Zaki MH, Wysocka M, et al. The role for interleukin-12 therapy of cutaneous T cell lymphoma. Ann N Y Acad Sci 2001;941:177–84.
33. Zaki MH, Wysocka M, Everetts SE, et al. Synergistic enhancement of cell-mediated immunity by interleukin-12 plus interleukin-2: basis for therapy of cutaneous T cell lymphoma. J Invest Dermatol 2002;118(2):366–71.
34. Mizutani N, Goto-Koshino Y, Tsuboi M, et al. Evaluation of CD25-positive cells in relation to the subtypes and prognoses in various lymphoid tumours in dogs. Vet Immunol Immunopathol 2016;173:39–43.
35. Lowenthal JW, Zubler RH, Nabholz M, et al. Similarities between interleukin-2 receptor number and affinity on activated B and T lymphocytes. Nature 1985; 315(6021):669–72.
36. Talpur R, Jones DM, Alencar AJ, et al. CD25 expression is correlated with histological grade and response to denileukin diftitox in cutaneous T-cell lymphoma. J Invest Dermatol 2006;126(3):575–83.
37. Fujiwara S, Muroi K, Tatara R, et al. Clinical features of de novo CD25-positive follicular lymphoma. Leuk Lymphoma 2014;55(2):307–13.
38. Chimura N, Kondo N, Shibata S, et al. Gene transcription analysis in lesional skin of canine epitheliotropic cutaneous lymphoma using quantitative real-time RT-PCR. Vet Immunol Immunopathol 2011;144(3):329–36.
39. Wilcock BP, Yager JA. The behavior of epidermotropic lymphoma in twenty-five dogs. Can Vet J 1989;30(9):754–6.
40. Mineshige T, Kawarai S, Yauchi T, et al. Cutaneous epitheliotropic T-cell lymphoma with systemic dissemination in a dog. J Vet Diagn Invest 2016;28(3): 327–31.
41. Fink-Puches R, Zenahlik P, Back B, et al. Primary cutaneous lymphomas: applicability of current classification schemes (European Organization for Research and Treatment of Cancer, World Health Organization) based on clinicopathologic features observed in a large group of patients. Blood 2002;99(3):800–5.
42. Willemze R, Kerl H, Sterry W, et al. EORTC classification for primary cutaneous lymphomas: a proposal from the cutaneous lymphoma study group of the European Organization for Research and Treatment of Cancer. Blood 1997; 90(1):354–71.
43. Guitart J, Martinez-Escala ME, Subtil A, et al. Primary cutaneous aggressive epidermotropic cytotoxic T-cell lymphomas: reappraisal of a provisional entity in the 2016 WHO classification of cutaneous lymphomas. Mod Pathol 2017;30(5): 761–72.
44. Laprais A, Olivry T. Is CCNU (lomustine) valuable for treatment of cutaneous epitheliotropic lymphoma in dogs? A critically appraised topic. BMC Vet Res 2017; 13(1):61.

45. Iwamoto KS, Bennett LR, Norman A, et al. Linoleate produces remission in canine mycosis fungoides. Cancer Lett 1992;64(1):17–22.
46. White SD, Rosychuk RA, Scott KV, et al. Use of isotretinoin and etretinate for the treatment of benign cutaneous neoplasia and cutaneous lymphoma in dogs. J Am Vet Med Assoc 1993;202(3):387–91.
47. Vail DM, Kravis LD, Cooley AJ, et al. Preclinical trial of doxorubicin entrapped in sterically stabilized liposomes in dogs with spontaneously arising malignant tumors. Cancer Chemother Pharmacol 1997;39(5):410–6.
48. Morges MA, Burton JH, Saba CF, et al. Phase II evaluation of VDC-1101 in canine cutaneous T-cell lymphoma. J Vet Intern Med 2014;28(5):1569–74.
49. De Clercq E. Tanovea(R) for the treatment of lymphoma in dogs. Biochem Pharmacol 2018;154:265–9.
50. Domenico S, Lyndsay K, Bo L, et al. Total skin electron therapy as treatment for epitheliotropic lymphoma in a dog. Vet Dermatol 2017;28(2):e65.
51. De Mello SC, Valli VEO, Selting KA, et al. Immunohistochemical detection of retinoid receptors in tumors from 30 dogs diagnosed with cutaneous lymphoma. J Vet Intern Med 2010;24(5):1112–7.
52. Gormley RH, Hess SD, Anand D, et al. Primary cutaneous aggressive epidermotropic CD8+ T-cell lymphoma. J Am Acad Dermatol 2010;62(2):300–7.
53. Nofal A, Abdel-Mawla MY, Assaf M, et al. Primary cutaneous aggressive epidermotropic CD8+ T-cell lymphoma: proposed diagnostic criteria and therapeutic evaluation. J Am Acad Dermatol 2012;67(4):748–59.
54. Kisseberth WC, Murahari S, London CA, et al. Evaluation of the effects of histone deacetylase inhibitors on cells from canine cancer cell lines. Am J Vet Res 2008; 69(7):938–45.
55. Mann BS, Johnson JR, He K, et al. Vorinostat for treatment of cutaneous manifestations of advanced primary cutaneous T-cell lymphoma. Clin Cancer Res 2007; 13(8):2318–22.
56. Fontaine J, Heimann M, Day MJ. Cutaneous epitheliotropic T-cell lymphoma in the cat: a review of the literature and five new cases. Vet Dermatol 2011;22(5): 454–61.
57. Legendre AM, Becker PU. Feline skin lymphoma: characterization of tumor and identification of tumor-stimulating serum factor(s). Am J Vet Res 1979;40(12): 1805–7.
58. Wood C, Almes K, Bagladi-Swanson M, et al. Sezary syndrome in a cat. J Am Anim Hosp Assoc 2008;44(3):144–8.
59. Tobey JC, Houston DM, Breur GJ, et al. Cutaneous T-cell lymphoma in a cat. J Am Vet Med Assoc 1994;204(4):606–9.
60. Caciolo PL, Nesbitt GH, Patnaik AK, et al. Cutaneous lymphosarcoma in the cat: a report of nine cases. J Am Anim Hosp Assoc 1984;20:491–6.
61. Jackson ML, Wood SL, Misra V, et al. Immunohistochemical identification of B and T lymphocytes in formalin-fixed, paraffin-embedded feline lymphosarcomas: relation to feline leukemia virus status, tumor site, and patient age. Can J Vet Res 1996;60(3):199–204.
62. Neta M, Naigamwalla D, Bienzle D. Perforin expression in feline epitheliotropic cutaneous lymphoma. J Vet Diagn Invest 2008;20(6):831–5.
63. Caciolo PL, Hayes AA, Patnaik AK, et al. A case of mycosis fungoides in a cat and literature review. J Am Anim Hosp Assoc 1983;19:505–12.
64. Baker JL, Scott DW. Mycosis fungoides in two cats. J Am Anim Hosp Assoc 1989; 25:97–101.

65. Gilbert S, Affolter VK, Gross TL, et al. Clinical, morphological and immunohisto-chemical characterization of cutaneous lymphocytosis in 23 cats. Vet Dermatol 2004;15(1):3–12.
66. Pariser MS, Gram DW. Feline cutaneous lymphocytosis: case report and summary of the literature. J Feline Med Surg 2014;16(9):758–63.
67. Affolter VK, Gross TL, Moore PF. Indolent cutaneous T-cell lymphoma presenting as cutaneous lymphocytosis in dogs. Vet Dermatol 2009;20(5–6):577–85.

Assessing Quality of Life for Pets with Dermatologic Disease and Their Owners

Chiara Noli, DVM

KEYWORDS

- Quality of life • Skin disease • Dog • Cat

KEY POINTS

- Quality of life (QoL) is a term used to evaluate general well-being, and it is defined as "the degree to which an individual enjoys his or her life." In medicine, QoL is often assessed in terms of how it is negatively affected by disease.
- In canine dermatology, 3 research groups have developed questionnaires for QoL assessment in dogs with dermatologic conditions, 2 being limited to canine atopic dermatitis, and 1 applicable to all skin conditions. One questionnaire was developed and validated in cats with dermatologic diseases.
- There usually is an inverse correlation between QoL and pruritus.
- In most studies in which QoL was evaluated before and after a therapeutic intervention, it usually improves quantitatively less than clinical parameters (pruritus, skin lesions), possibly as a consequence of the burden of treatment.
- It is thus important to measure QoL in parallel with clinical parameters in clinical trials.

INTRODUCTION

Quality of life (QoL) is a term used to evaluate general well-being, and it is defined as "the degree to which an individual enjoys his or her life." In medicine, QoL is often assessed in terms of how it is negatively affected by disease.

QoL evaluation is considered to be one of the main outcomes in human clinical trials,[1] and it is used frequently in primary care practice.[2] QoL has been studied and evaluated in small animal medicine only over the past few years. Recently, QoL surveys have been developed for various diseases in dogs, such as cardiopathies,[1] spinal cord injuries,[3] osteoarthritis,[4] chronic pain,[5] cancer,[6] kidney disease,[7] and inflammatory bowel disease.[8]

The author has nothing to disclose.
Servizi Dermatologici Veterinari, Strada Bedale della Ressia 2, Peveragno, Cuneo 12016, Italy
E-mail address: info@dermatologiaveterinaria.it

QUESTIONNAIRES EVALUATING QUALITY OF LIFE IN DERMATOLOGIC PATIENTS: THE HUMAN PERSPECTIVE

Skin diseases include a broad range of disorders in humans, and for some people, these conditions lead to psychological stress and reduced QoL. Many studies have evaluated QoL in people with skin disease.[9] Widely used questionnaires on the impact of dermatologic diseases on QoL are the Skindex[10] and the Dermatology Life Quality Index (DLQI).[11] Questionnaires have been published for specific dermatitides, such as psoriasis, acne, urticaria, onychomycosis, and leg ulcers.[9] For children (Children Dermatology Life Quality Index, CDLQI)[12] and infants (Childhood Atopic Dermatitis Impact Scale[13] and Infants Dermatitis Quality of Life Index[14] [IDQOL]) special questionnaires have also been published, which are usually compiled by parents or caregivers. Skin conditions not only have an important influence on the patients' lives, but can also affect the life of the people in the same household, sometimes more than that of the patients themselves. For this reason, a Family Dermatology Quality of Life Index (FDLQI)[15,16] and a Dermatitis Family Impact Questionnaire (DFI) were also developed.[17]

QUESTIONNAIRES VALIDATED FOR CANINE SKIN DISEASES

In spite of the obvious fact that itch and pain caused by dermatologic conditions can have an impact on QoL of affected animals, until 2010 there were only 2 studies evaluating QoL in dogs with skin disease. In 1 of these studies, the dogs represented a control group.[18] In the other study, allergic dogs were treated with a 0.025% budesonide leave-on-conditioner and evaluated for lesions, pruritus, and QoL by means of a nonvalidated scale.[19] Since then, 2 research groups have developed and validated questionnaires for QoL assessment in dogs with dermatologic conditions, the first being limited to canine atopic dermatitis,[20,21] and the second applicable to all skin conditions.[22,23]

The main questionnaires on the impact of dermatologic diseases on QoL used in human medicine are the Skindex (and subsequent developments)[10] and the Dermatology Life Quality Index (DLQI) (and subsequent developments).[11] Interestingly, the questionnaire developed by Favrot and colleagues[20] took the Skindex as an example, while the questionnaire developed by Noli and colleagues[22] was inspired by the DLQI.

There are several differences between these 2 questionnaires. The questionnaire developed by Favrot and colleagues[20] is composed of several statements, to which the owner should declare his or her agreement or disagreement. Evaluation of each item is thus performed by assigning a score to each statement from 0 (strongly disagree) to 4 (strongly agree). The initial version of this questionnaire comprised 16 questions related to the QoL of the owner, and 14 to the QoL of the dog, followed by 6 related to the treatment of CAD in a subsequent publication.[21] Part of these questions reflected those established and validated for the assessment of QoL of children affected by atopic dermatitis and that of their parents. The aim of the other questions was to evaluate the impact of the disease on the overall benefit of pet ownership, and some were related to the activities of the dog and its well-being. In this questionnaire, the lifestyle of the dog (eg, indoor vs outdoor, urban vs rural) was also considered, as it has been previously observed that dogs living in a rural or suburban environment have higher QoL,[24] and owners of diseased dogs living mainly indoors may have a lower QoL because of the constant disturbance by their pet's disease. Favrot also determined that owners with a very close relationship to their dogs considered the impact on their QoL higher.

The questionnaire by Favrot and colleagues[20] was evaluated for content validity by asking veterinarians, nurses, and pet owners to assess whether the statements were adequate and relevant. Construct validity was evaluated by calculating the correlation between answers to the overall assessment questions and the lesional scores (CADESI-03). There were 2 overall assessment questions, 1 question aiming at determining the impact of the disease on the owner's QoL and the other on the dog's QoL; the actual 30 + item questionnaire followed. Unfortunately no correlation was determined between the whole questionnaire and lesional or pruritus scores. After statistical evaluation of the answers to the single questions and the significance of each for the assessment of QoL, the authors concluded that several questions could be eliminated and proposed a shorter 15-item questionnaire for further studies. To the author's knowledge, there is only 1 published clinical study that used this questionnaire until now.[25]

The other questionnaire developed by Noli and coworkers[22] comprises questions to which owners can answer "none - a little - quite a bit - very much," with scores ranging respectively from 0 to 3. The content of the questions was derived from detailed preliminary ethnographic interviews with owners of dogs affected with severe skin conditions. These were free-form conversations in which owners were encouraged to describe how their dog's disease was disturbing their QoL and that of their pets. The main areas identified in which the dog's life could be disturbed by the disease were: sleep, eating, behavior, play or work, relationship with owners and other dogs, and disturbance caused by administration of therapies. Also, the main areas identified in which the owner's life could be disturbed by their dog's disease were: practical problems (eg, more cleaning or cooking), time loss, psychological aspects (eg, feeling of guilt, frustration, or shame), disturbance of the normal family life and of interpersonal relationships within or outside the family, disturbance of sleep, disturbance in the relationship with their dog, financial expenditure, and reduced dog's working performances. From an initial 19-item version, 4 irrelevant or redundant questions were removed, and a final 15-item questionnaire was published comprising 1 question on the general severity of the disease, 7 questions dealing with the QoL of dogs (QoL1), and 7 questions dealing with the QoL of the owners (QoL2). This questionnaire is now available as supporting information on the Veterinary Dermatology Web page.[26] Criterion-related validity was evaluated by comparing QoL1 and QoL2 scores with CADESI-03 and with pruritus assessed by means of a validated Visual Analogue Scale. Construct validity was determined by calculating the correlation of the owner-perceived general severity (question 1) with QoL1 and QoL2. Furthermore this questionnaire was also tested for repeatability and for sensitivity to capture differences between a healthy and a diseased population and improvement after treatment. Several articles have been published since using this questionnaire for the evaluation of treatment success in parallel with clinical scores.[27–31]

Very recently, another research group has been working on developing and validating a new questionnaire on QoL and treatment success (TS) in dogs with atopic dermatitis, using methodology informed by the US Food and Drug Administration (FDA) questionnaire development guidance.[32–34] In the development phase of this new questionnaire, owners of dogs with allergic dermatitis were interviewed, and the most important reported signs of allergy were itching, biting, licking, and sleep disturbance. Owners reported impact on emotional well-being, such as empathy and sadness, as well as on finances, sleep, and daily routine. Besides taking TS into account, this questionnaire differs by the previous ones in that in 2 studies it was completed by owners at home by means of an app on a smartphone (PicorCan, ItchTracker).[35,36]

THE IMPACT OF CANINE ATOPIC DERMATITIS ON QUALITY OF LIFE

As mentioned previously, in their validation process, both questionnaires developed by Favrot and colleagues[20] and by Noli and colleagues[22] were administered to owners of atopic dogs, in which CADESI-03 and VAS pruritus scores were also measured. In the study by Noli and colleagues, correlation between QoL and pruritus scores was good and significant, indicating that pruritus has an important impact on QoL of dogs and their owners. On the other hand, correlation was not as good between QoL and CADESI-03, confirming that the sole evaluation of lesional improvement in trials is not sufficient, and that the success of a therapeutic intervention, as experienced by owners and pets, is determined by other factors besides clinical improvement. It is clear that clinical scores alone do not reflect the disease experienced by the patient, as they do not take into account any impairment of QoL. To a similar conclusion came Favrot and colleagues,[20] who reported correlations between "overall assessment questions" and CADESI-03, but "never close to full concordance unity, emphasizing that the different parameters measure different facets of the same phenomenon and are consequently all useful to evaluate the severity of the disease."

In the study by Linek and Favrot, 73% of the owners considered that atopic dermatitis had an impact on the QoL of their animals, and the higher the CADESI and the pruritus, the higher was the impact on QoL.[21] The areas of the dogs' lives that were most impaired by atopic dermatitis in the questionnaire by Noli and colleagues[22] were behavioral or mood changes, playing/working activities, and the burden of administering treatment. In contrast, Linek and Favrot judged sleep disturbance to be an important factor, while playing was not strongly affected.[21] These differences could be determined by the different questionnaire structure or wording, as well as by different lifestyles in the 2 study populations, which came from Italy and Germany/Austria, respectively. In both studies, meals were not greatly affected.

In the study by Linek and Favrot, 48% of the owners considered that atopic dermatitis had an impact on their own QoL, and the higher the CADESI and the closer the relationship to the animals, the higher was the impact on QoL.[21] The areas of the owners' life that were most impaired in both studies were increased expenditure, time loss, and emotional and physical distress, while family activities and intrafamily relationships were less involved.

Recently, the new questionnaire on QoL and TS developed by Wright and colleagues was used to analyze the association between pruritus (before and after oclacitinib treatment) and QoL of dogs and owners.[34] This study observed a significant association between pruritus and QoL, in that QoL decreased as pruritus increased. However, this observation was not confirmed by a subsequent study that used lokivetmab as antipruritic agent,[36] in that the dogs' QoL scores did not improve as pruritus decreased. However, in the 2 studies, the dogs included were very different; dogs treated with oclacitinib were presenting for acute pruritus and were not on any prior therapy, while those treated with lokivetmab were severe chronic cases that had not responded to any previous medication.

THE USE OF QUALITY OF LIFE QUESTIONNAIRES IN CLINICAL STUDIES

There are by now several studies in veterinary dermatology using QoL as a parameter for the assessment of a treatment intervention in dogs with atopic dermatitis[19,23,25,27–29,31,37] or other dermatologic conditions.[30]

The study by Ahlstrom and colleagues[19] used a nonvalidated owner-assessed 10 cm long visual analogue scale with descriptors that ranged from 0 (=distracted, not usual self, uncomfortable, unhappy, not playing or attentive) to 10 (=bright, alert, comfortable, happy, attentive, playful, responsive to family), and evaluated QoL in atopic dogs treated with barazone. This study also evaluated lesions and pruritus before and after intervention. Interestingly, QoL improvement was significant, albeit quantitatively inferior to that of lesions and pruritus, highlighting the need for QoL assessment as an extra tool in the evaluation of treatment interventions. Similar observations were made by subsequent studies using different questionnaires.[20,27,28,31]

The study by Cosgrove and colleagues[37] used a self-designed nonvalidated questionnaire derived from those developed by Favrot and colleagues[20] and Linek and Favrot.[21] In this study, QoL was assessed only once after dogs had been treated long term with oclacitinib.[37] Although this particular questionnaire partly related to and was biased in favor of the treatment molecule oclacitinib ("Previous treatments have not resolved my dog's condition and are time consuming" or "Confident that the current treatment (ocalcitinib) is effective" or "Quality of life after oclacitinib"), it identified aspects of the dogs' and of the owners' lives that were disturbed by the disease, in agreement with the other validated assessment tools, in particular worsening of the dogs' behavior, decrease of playing activities, sleep disturbance of dogs and owners, as well as burden of veterinary consultations were reported by 58% to 98% of the owners, depending on the item.

The study by Litzlbauer and colleagues[25] evaluated QoL in atopic dogs undergoing treatment with recombinant feline interferon omega and is thus far the only study that used the questionnaire developed by Favrot and colleagues.[20] Concurrent medication was permitted. Although clinical lesions improved by 36% to 62% (depending on the treatment group), and pruritus improved by 24% to 36%, QoL scores improved only by about 10%.

All other studies used the questionnaire developed by Noli and colleagues,[22,23] and besides clinical parameters (pruritus or lesions), assessed QoL of dogs and of their owners before and after a therapeutic intervention. Three of these[23,27,29] were used in atopic dogs, 2 in dogs with food allergy,[28,31] and one in dogs with otitis.[30]

One study evaluated the impact of an essential fatty acid supplement, versus a placebo, as a ciclosporin-sparing agent in 2 groups of dogs whose allergic disease was under control with ciclosporin.[29] QoL was assessed before and at the end of the study, together with lesions (CADESI-03) and pruritus (VAS). In this study, lesional and pruritus scores improved significantly more in the supplemented group compared with placebo, but surprisingly, QoL score improvement was similar in both groups (about 30%), possibly reflecting the advantages of being included in a controlled study (eg, free medications and veterinary consultations).

In other studies, QoL of dogs (QoL1) and that of owners (QoL2) were assessed separately. One of these,[23] used for the validation of the questionnaire, reported a higher mean improvement for QoL1 compared with QoL2, and analysis of the single questions clearly highlighted that the therapeutic interventions necessary to keep the pet's dermatologic conditions under control did impact negatively on the owners' and the dogs' QoL (**Fig. 1**). It is worth noting that in this study dogs undergoing any kind of therapy were enrolled, including interventions that are expensive (eg, ciclosporin) or labor intensive (eg, shampoo).

In another study,[27] however, treatment was made easy, as dogs received just 1 or 2 daily palatable capsules, which were free of cost for the owner. Interestingly in this study, the 2 QoL subclusters improved to a similar extent in response to treatment, maybe confirming that an inexpensive and nonlabor-intensive treatment will also improve the owner's QoL.

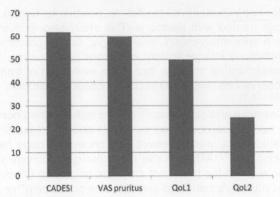

Fig. 1. Improvement of lesional scores (CADESI), pruritus, dog's QoL (QoL1) and owner's QoL (QoL2) in dogs with atopic dermatitis after treatment. It is evident that QoL improvement does not mirror lesional and pruritus improvement, particularly for the owners. (*Data from* Noli C, Colombo S, Cornegliani L, et al. Quality of life of dogs with skin disease and of their owners - part 2: administration of a questionnaire in various skin diseases and correlation to efficacy of therapy. Vet Dermatol 2011;22:344–51.)

This observation was strongly confirmed by a recent study on assessment of QoL in dogs affected with otitis and undergoing different therapeutic interventions.[30] In this study, fifty client-owned dogs were randomly divided into two groups and treated for 2 weeks. One group was treated with a medicated gel twice 1 week apart by the veterinarian, with no involvement of owners in the treatment procedures. The other group was treated daily by the owners with medicated ear drops and twice-weekly cleanings. In all dogs, clinical parameters, such as pruritus and ear lesions, improved, with no difference between groups. However, there was a significantly higher improvement of dogs' and owners' QoL in the first group compared with the second group, demonstrating that the administration of treatments can have a negative impact on QoL of dogs and owners (**Fig. 2**). This observation confirms the need of QoL evaluation, together with the assessment of clinical parameters in clinical studies. It is also worth mentioning that QoL improvements in this study were extremely high, up to 77% for QoL1 on day 28, much higher than that observed for interventions in atopic or food allergic dogs. This discrepancy could be attributable to the nature of the disease or of the interventions and their impact on the patient and owner.

The other 2 studies evaluating QoL in dogs with food allergy and therapeutic therapy gave results in line with those published for atopic dermatitis.[28,31]

The new questionnaire developed by Wright and colleagues was used in clinical studies that used oclacitinib or lokivetmab to relieve pruritus and signs of atopic dermatitis in dogs.[34–36] In 1 open[35] study on 30 cases, pruritus improved by 54%, the owners' QoL by 23%, and the dogs' QoL by 52%, in agreement with previous observations using a different questionnnaire.[27] Surprisingly, in another study using lokivetmab, parallel to pruritus decrease, only the owners' QoL improved, and the dogs' QoL remained essentially the same.[36] This finding is unusual and in contrast with all previously reported studies, and may be explained with the high level of QoL that the patients already had at the beginning of the study, or with a particular patient population used in this study. More investigations are needed for the evaluation and validation of this new QoL and TS assessment tool.

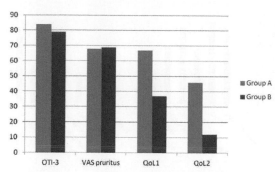

Fig. 2. Improvement of lesional scores (OTI-3), pruritus, dog's QoL (QoL1), and owner's QoL (QoL2) in dogs with otitis treated with 2 different interventions (group A and group B). Although there is no difference in clinical efficacy between the 2 products, there is a great difference in QoL improvement. (*Data from* Noli C, Sartori R, Cena T. Impact of a terbinafine–florfenicol–betamethasone acetate otic gel on the quality of life of dogs with acute otitis externa and their owners. Vet Dermatol 2017;28:386-e90.)

QUALITY OF LIFE ASSESSMENT IN FELINE DERMATOLOGY

There are only a few studies proposing QoL assessments in cats[38] for degenerative joint disease,[39] cardiopathies,[40] feline infectious peritonitis,[41] diabetes mellitus[42] and chemotherapy for lymphoma,[43] and skin disease.[44–46]

A feline version of questionnaire for the assessment of QoL of cats with skin disease was developed and validated,[44] with a format similar to that used for dogs[22] (eg, with one subset for animals and one for their owners). Twenty long interviews were administered to owners of cats with skin disease, for the identification of areas of the cats' and the owners' life that could be negatively influenced by the pet's skin disease. Interestingly, in the development of this questionnaire, items such as physical uneasiness or discomfort because of the cats' clinical condition were less important for cat than for dog owners (cats obviously have less dramatic skin diseases than dogs). On the other hand, items such as stress due to administration of therapies and to visits to the veterinarian were more important for cats and their owners than for dogs and their owners, highlighting the fact that treating cats is certainly more difficult and a bigger source of psychological stress than treating dogs (**Fig. 3**).

In its validating procedure, this preliminary questionnaire was used in a clinical study assessing the efficacy of liquid ciclosporin in cats with allergic dermatitis.[45] Thirty-two cats were treated with a mean ciclosporin dosage of 7.3 mg/kg/d and followed for 3 months. As in dogs, pruritus scores significantly and inversely correlated with QoL. In this study, lesional (SCORFAD) improvement was good/excellent in 91.6% of cases, pruritus in 81.5%, albeit QoL only in 56.25%. Improvement of SCORFAD and pruritus were statistically significant, but not QoL. A detailed analysis of the 2 subsets QoL1 and QoL2 determined that treatment administration and veterinary visits had a great impact on QoL of cats and of their owners.

The feline version of the QoL questionnaire was subsequently used in a multicenter randomized, blinded, methylprednisolone-controlled study aiming at the determination of the efficacy of oclacitinib in feline allergic dermatitis.[46] Contrary to the previous study, a significant improvement of pruritus and lesions (54%–69% depending on the parameter and on the treatment group) was associated with a significant improvement of QoL, albeit by a smaller extent (21%–25%).

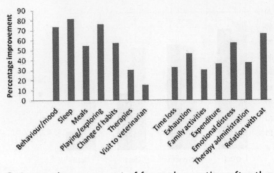

Fig. 3. Percentage QoL score improvement of for each question after therapy in 37 cats with allergic dermatitis. The 7 bars to the left relate to the cat's QoL, and the 7 bars to the right to the owner's QoL. It is evident that aspects related to therapy administration and visits to the veterinarian improve less than other items. (*Data from* Noli C, Borio S, Varina A, et al. Development and validation of a questionnaire to evaluate the quality of life of cats with skin disease and their owners, and its use in 185 cats with skin disease. Vet Dermatol 2016;27:247-e58.)

SUMMARY

QoL is a term used to evaluate general well-being, and is defined as "the degree to which an individual enjoys his or her life." In medicine, QoL is often assessed in terms of how it is negatively affected by disease. In canine dermatology, 2 research groups have developed and validated questionnaires for QoL assessment in dogs with dermatologic conditions, the first being limited to canine atopic dermatitis, and the second applicable to all skin conditions. A third group is currently working on the validation of a different QoL questionnaire coupled with a treatment success assessment tool. In general, there is an inverse correlation between QoL and pruritus. There are by now several studies in veterinary dermatology using QoL as a parameter for the assessment of a treatment intervention in dogs and cats with dermatologic diseases, in particular canine atopic dermatitis. In most of these studies, following a therapeutic intervention, QoL usually improves quantitatively less than clinical parameters (pruritus, skin lesions). This observation can represent the consequence of the burden of treatment and underlines the importance of measuring QoL in parallel with clinical parameters in clinical trials.

ACKNOWLEDGMENTS

Part of this article is taken from: Noli C. Quality of life in veterinary dermatology. proceedings scientific session of the North American Veterinary Dermatology Forum. Nashville, TN, 2015: p. 232–6; with permission.

REFERENCES

1. Freeman LM, Rush JE, Farabaugh AE. Development and evaluation of a questionnaire for assessing health-related quality of life in dogs with cardiac disease. J Am Vet Med Assoc 2005;226:1864–8.

2. Calvert MJ, Freemantle N. Use of health-related quality of life in prescribing research. Part 1: why evaluate health-related quality of life? J Clin Pharm Ther 2003;28:513–21.

3. Budke CM, Levine JM, Kerwin SC, et al. Evaluation of a questionnaire for obtaining owner-perceived, weighted quality-of-life assessments for dogs with spinal cord injuries. J Am Vet Med Assoc 2008;233:925–30.

4. Hielm-Björkman AK, Rita H, Tulamo RM. Psychometric testing of the Helsinki chronic pain index by completion of a questionnaire in Finnish by owners of dogs with chronic signs of pain caused by osteoarthritis. Am J Vet Res 2009; 70:727–34.

5. Wiseman-Orr ML, Nolan AM, Reid J, et al. Development of a questionnaire to measure the effects of chronic pain on health-related quality of life in dogs. Am J Vet Res 2004;65:1077–84.

6. Lynch S, Savary-Bataille K, Leeuw B, et al. Development of a questionnaire assessing health-related quality-of-life in dogs and cats with cancer. Vet Comp Oncol 2011;9:172–82.

7. Yearley JH, Hancock DD, Mealey KL. Survival time, lifespan, and quality of life in dogs with idiopathic Fanconi syndrome. J Am Vet Med Assoc 2004;225:377–83.

8. Craven M, Simpson JW, Ridyard AE, et al. Canine inflammatory bowel disease: retrospective analysis of diagnosis and outcome in 80 cases (1995–2002). J Small Anim Pract 2004;45:336–42.

9. Finlay AY. Quality of life measurement in dermatology: a practical guide. Br J Dermatol 1997;136:305–14.

10. Chren MM, Lasek RJ, Quinn LM, et al. Skindex, a quality-of-life measure for patients with skin disease: reliability, validity, and responsiveness. J Invest Dermatol 1996;107:707–13.

11. Finlay AY, Khan GK. Dermatology life quality index (DLQI): a simple practical measure for routine clinical use. Clin Exp Dermatol 1994;19:210–6.

12. Lewis-Jones MS, Finlay AY. The children's dermatology life quality index (CDLQI): initial validation and practical use. Br J Dermatol 1995;132:942–9.

13. Chamlin SL, Lai JS, Cella D, et al. Childhood atopic dermatitis impact scale: reliability, discriminative and concurrent validity, and responsiveness. Arch Dermatol 2007;143:768–72.

14. Lewis-Jones MS, Finlay AY, Dykes PJ. The infant's dermatitis quality of life index. Br J Dermatol 2001;144:104–10.

15. Basra MKA, Sue-Ho R, Finley AY. The family dermatology life quality index: measuring the secondary impact of skin disease. Br J Dermatol 2007;156: 528–38 [Erratum appears in Br J Dermatol 2007;156:791].

16. Basra MKA, Edmunds O, Salek MS, et al. Measurement of family impact of skin disease: further validation of the family dermatology life quality index (FDLQI). J Eur Acad Dermatol Venereol 2008;22:813–21.

17. Lawson V, Lewis-Jones MS, Finlay AY, et al. The family impact of childhood atopic dermatitis: the Dermatitis Family Impact questionnaire. Br J Dermatol 1998;138: 107–13.

18. Yazbek KVB, Fantoni T. Validity of a health-related quality-of-life scale for dogs with signs of pain secondary to cancer. J Am Vet Med Assoc 2005;226:1354–8.

19. Ahlstrom LA, Mason KV, Mills PC. Barazone decreases skin lesions and pruritus and increases quality of life in dogs with atopic dermatitis: a randomized, blinded, placebo-controlled trial. J Vet Pharmacol Ther 2010;33:573–82.

20. Favrot C, Linek M, Mueller R, et al. Development of a questionnaire to assess the impact of atopic dermatitis on health-related quality of life of affected dogs and their owners. Vet Dermatol 2010;21:64–70.

21. Linek M, Favrot C. Impact of canine atopic dermatitis on the health-related quality of life of affected dogs and quality of life of their owners. Vet Dermatol 2010;21: 456–62.
22. Noli C, Minafò G, Galzerano M. Quality of life of dogs with skin disease and their owners - part 1: development and validation of a questionnaire. Vet Dermatol 2011;22:335–43.
23. Noli C, Colombo S, Cornegliani L, et al. Quality of life of dogs with skin disease and of their owners - part 2: administration of a questionnaire in various skin diseases and correlation to efficacy of therapy. Vet Dermatol 2011;22:344–51.
24. Wojciechowska JI, Hewson CJ, Stryhn H, et al. Evaluation of a questionnaire regarding nonphysical aspects of quality of life in sick and healthy dogs. Am J Vet Res 2005;66:1461–7.
25. Litzlbauer P, Weber K, Mueller RS. Oral and subcutaneous therapy of canine atopic dermatitis with recombinant feline interferon omega. Cytokine 2014;66: 54–9.
26. Available at: http://onlinelibrary.wiley.com/doi/10.1111/j.1365-3164.2011.00956.x/suppinfo. Accessed May 19, 2018.
27. Noli C, Della Valle MF, Miolo A, et al. Efficacy of ultra-micronized palmitoylethanolamide in canine atopic dermatitis: an open-label multi-centre study. Vet Dermatol 2015;26:432–40.
28. Maina E, Cox E. A double-blind, randomized, placebo controlled trial of the efficacy, quality of life and safety of food allergen-specific sublingual immunotherapy in client owned dogs with adverse food reactions: a small pilot study. Vet Dermatol 2016;27:361-e91.
29. Müller RM, Linek M, Löwenstein C, et al. Evaluation of cyclosporine-sparing effects of polyunsaturated fatty acids in the treatment of canine atopic dermatitis. Vet J 2016;210:77–81.
30. Noli C, Sartori R, Cena T. Impact of a terbinafine–florfenicol–betamethasone acetate otic gel on the quality of life of dogs with acute otitis externa and their owners. Vet Dermatol 2017;28:386-e90.
31. Matricoti I, Noli C. An open label clinical trial to evaluate the utility of a hydrolysed fish and rice starch elimination diet for the diagnosis of adverse food reactions in dogs. Vet Dermatol 2018. [Epub ahead of print].
32. Wright A, Tatlock S, Wells J, et al. Development of the canine dermatitis quality of life and treatment satisfaction questionnaire: a tool for clinical practice. Proceedings NAVDF (abstract). Vet Dermatol 2017;28:453.
33. Wright A, Tatlock S, Wells JR, et al. Psychometric evaluation and interpretation of change of the canine dermatitis quality of life and treatment satisfaction questionnaire (CDQoL-TSQ). proceedings ESVD (abstract). Vet Dermatol 2017;28:553.
34. Wright A, Cooper S, Pavlock A. Association of administration of oclacitinib with improvement of quality of life of acutely pruritic dogs and their owners in 7 days (abstract). Vet Dermatol 2018;7. https://doi.org/10.1111/vde.12546.
35. Wright A, Alaman C, Holland R. Preliminary results from a mobile app monitoring canine pruritus and quality of life in dogs prescribed oclacitinib (abstract). Vet Dermatol 2018;4. https://doi.org/10.1111/vde.12546.
36. Nguyen TS, Simpson B, L'Estrange R, et al. Progress report from an early experience program involving atopic dogs treated with lokivetmab reaching 30 days post injection using a mobile application monitoring pruritus and dog and owner quality of life (QoL). (abstract) Proceedings from the Australian Small Animal Veterinarians Innovation, Research and Development Symposium. Australian Vet Association Annual Conference Brisbane, Queensland 2018;9–10.

37. Cosgrove SB, Cleaver DM, King VL, et al. Long-term compassionate use of ocla-citinib in dogs with atopic and allergic skin disease: safety, efficacy and quality of life. Vet Dermatol 2015;26:171-e35.
38. Tatlock S, Gober M, Williamson N, et al. Development and preliminary psycho-metric evaluation of an owner-completed measure of feline quality of life. Vet J 2017;228:22–32.
39. Benito J, Gruen ME, Thomson A, et al. Owner-assessed indices of quality of life in cats and the relationship to the presence of degenerative joint disease. J Feline Med Surg 2012;14:863–70.
40. Freeman LM, Rush JE, Oyama MA, et al. Development and evaluation of a ques-tionnaire for assessment of health-related quality of life in cats with cardiac dis-ease. J Am Vet Med Assoc 2012;240:1188–93.
41. Fischer Y, Ritz S, Weber K, et al. Randomized, placebo controlled study of the effect of propentofylline on survival time and quality of life of cats with feline infec-tious peritonitis. J Vet Intern Med 2011;25:1270–6.
42. Niessen SJ, Powney S, Guitian J, et al. Evaluation of a quality-of-life tool for cats with diabetes mellitus. J Vet Intern Med 2010;24:1098–105.
43. Tzannes S, Hammond MF, Murphy S, et al. Owners 'perception of their cats' qual-ity of life during COP chemotherapy for lymphoma. J Feline Med Surg 2008;10: 73–81.
44. Noli C, Borio S, Varina A, et al. Development and validation of a questionnaire to evaluate the quality of life of cats with skin disease and their owners, and its use in 185 cats with skin disease. Vet Dermatol 2016;27:247-e58.
45. Noli C, Ortalda C, Galzerano M. L'utilizzo della ciclosporina in formulazione liquida (Atoplus gatto®) nel trattamento delle malattie allergiche feline. Veterina-ria (Cremona) 2014;28:15–22.
46. Noli C, Matricoti I, Schievano C. Efficacy of oclacitinib in allergic cats: a multicen-tric randomised, blinded, methylprednisolone-controlled study (abstract). Vet Dermatol 2017;28:548.

Feline Pemphigus Foliaceus

Diane E. Preziosi, DVM

KEYWORDS

- Pemphigus foliaceus • Cats • Felines • Autoimmune skin disease

KEY POINTS

- Pemphigus foliaceus presents as a largely symmetric pustular to crusting dermatosis that most commonly targets the face, ears, and feet, but can also affect the trunk and legs.
- Diagnosis is achieved through physical examination, cytology, ruling out other pustular/crusting disorders, and procuring proper biopsy samples for dermatopathology.
- The histopathology of pemphigus foliaceus in cats, although sharing many features seen in other species such as acantholytic keratinocytes within pustules, often features large numbers of mast cells within the dermis.
- Treatment recommendations have changed over time and reflect new knowledge on how cats metabolize prednisone versus prednisolone and how newer drugs such as cyclosporine may be useful for treating this autoimmune disease.

INTRODUCTION

Pemphigus foliaceus (PF) is the most common form of pemphigus seen in domestic cats as well as the most common autoimmune skin disorder in this species.[1] However, little is known about the exact adhesion molecule targeted in this species. Like most other animals, cats develop pustules that rupture easily to form crusts. Cats have a distribution pattern involving their head, ears, and paws, but the trunk can also be involved.[2–4] Although the clinical signs and cytology can be very suggestive, histopathology is needed to confirm the diagnosis. Treatment has evolved over the years as new knowledge about how cats metabolize prednisone has become known and new drugs have become available.

PATHOGENESIS

Pemphigus is a disease complex that affects many species—humans, dogs, cats, horses, goats—and it has recently been reported in a sheep.[5,6] In these species, the intercellular connections between keratinocytes within the stratum granulosum are attacked by immunoglobulins causing separation of the keratinocytes. When this happens, the keratinocytes are released from the underlying epidermal layers

The author has nothing to disclose.
Veterinary Specialists of Alaska, 3330 Fairbanks Street, Anchorage, AK 99503, USA
E-mail address: dermsurgak@aol.com

and round up. These keratinocytes have a darkly stained cytoplasm with an intact nucleus and are referred to "acantholytic keratinocytes" or "acantholytic cells." The desmosomal target is known in people and in dogs, but is unknown in cats. Inflammatory cells invade the epidermis, where the adhesion molecules are attacked and a pustule is formed.

So far there, has been no age, breed, or sex predilection identified in feline PF. In the largest retrospective study published to date involving 57 cats, the age at which cats can be affected ranged from less than 1 to 17 years with a median age of 5 years.[2] A recently presented study of 49 cats had similar results, reporting cats ranging in age from 5 months to 15 years with a median age of 6 years.[7] The underlying cause for PF in cats has not been determined in most cases, but the possibility of some cases being drug induced has been suggested. Drugs may directly induce PF by triggering proteolytic enzymes in the skin that attack the desmosomes leading to acantholysis.[8] Drug-induced PF has been reported in humans and dogs. Several cases have reportedly been due to methimazole, which looks identical on histopathology to non–drug-induced PF.[2,9] Other authors have reported cases possibly due to cimetidine, ampicillin, itraconazole/lime sulfur, and ipodate.[2,10–12] Cases of PF caused by drugs might develop lesions rapidly and could have an early age of onset, oral lesions, or a feature atypical to naturally occurring PF.[9] In drug-triggered PF, the drug stimulates the immune system to form autoantibodies against intercellular connections. This type of PF may go into remission when the drug is withdrawn or, in those individuals with a predisposition for autoimmune problems, the disease must receive treatment after drug withdrawal.[1] Most cases of feline PF have no known underlying trigger.

CLINICAL FEATURES

The earliest lesion of feline PF may be an erythematous macule.[13] However, the macular phase is rarely noted because the disease quickly enters the pustular phase. Unlike pustules caused by bacterial folliculitis, pustules caused by pemphigus span multiple hair follicles.[9] Pustules are fragile, thus transient, and become dried, honey-colored crusts.[13] The crusts can be irregular in shape and can coalesce.[14] Under the crusts can be intact, alopecic, flaky skin or more often erosions.[1–4] When the disease affects the nails and paws, there is paronychia with erosion to ulceration involving the nail beds, often with purulent exudate (**Fig. 1**). The pads are often scaly

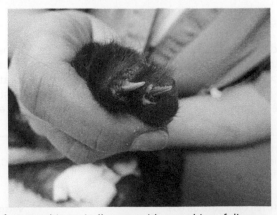

Fig. 1. Close-up of paronychia typically seen with pemphigus foliaceus.

with crusts at the edges.[1-4] One author feels that feline PF is the most common cause of feline nail fold and pad disease.[13]

In the 2 largest retrospective studies to date the most common areas affected were the pinna followed by the rest of the head/face, which included the periocular area, nose/muzzle, and chin[2,7] (**Fig. 2**). One study separated the muzzle and nares out statistically and found that they were involved in more than one-half of the cases[7] (**Fig. 3**). The next most commonly affected site was the paw (**Fig. 4**). The dorsal and ventral trunk areas were involved about one-half as frequently as the paws in 1 study,[2] and more frequently in another study with periareolar involvement noted in about one-quarter of the cases.[7] These sites were consistent with previous studies.[3,4] All studies agreed that the disease was bilaterally symmetric.[2-4,7] Systemic signs can be seen in some patients, including mild to moderate pruritus, lethargy, pyrexia, and less commonly anorexia, weight loss, and lymphadenopathy.[2-4] Lameness was sometimes noted when the nails and pads were severely affected.[2-4] Pruritus was seen in 66% to 80% of the cases in the 2 largest retrospective studies.[2,7]

The results of blood work were reported in 2 studies. Complete blood counts were run on a total of 35 cats. Leukocytosis, owing to neutrophilia, often eosinophilia, possibly lymphocytosis or lymphopenia, and monocytosis were found.[2,3] Serum biochemical profiles were performed on 33 cats and changes were usually mild and nonspecific. All cats tested for feline leukemia virus (3 cats) or both feline leukemia virus and feline immunodeficiency virus (18 cats) were negative.[2,3]

DIFFERENTIAL DIAGNOSES

Based on the clinical signs, other disease processes can be considered. This list includes diseases that can produce crusting and hair loss and include: pyoderma, superficial fungal dermatitis caused by *Trichophyton* spp., drug eruption, and allergy with secondary infection, as well as pemphigus erythematosus or herpes viral dermatitis if the lesions are confined to the head.[9]

DIAGNOSIS

It has been stated by 1 expert who has studied pemphigoid diseases extensively that there are 3 criteria that must be satisfied to make a diagnosis of PF:

1. Clinically—pustules that evolve to shallow erosions and crusts involving the face and feet;
2. Histopathologically—superficial epidermal or follicular pustules with neutrophils and acantholytic keratinocytes; and
3. Rule out other acantholytic neutrophilic pustular disorders, especially exfoliative-associated staphylococcal pyoderma and pustular dermatophytosis.[5]

If a cat presents with a crusting dermatosis of the face, ears, feet, or other areas, start looking for an intact pustule. Performing a Tzanck preparation is ideal. For this, a pustule is carefully ruptured with a small gauge needle and the contents are gently rolled on a slide. Standard stains can be used after that. A sample from a cat with PF will have many nondegenerate neutrophils along with variable numbers of acantholytic keratinocytes (**Fig. 5**). These are rounded immature keratinocytes from the stratum granulosum layer, about 4 times the size of a neutrophil or larger with a variably sized nucleus. The whole cell stains a dark bluish-purple using a standard Diff-quick stain commonly used in most general practices.[1,2,14] This finding is in contrast with a pustule owing to bacterial folliculitis that typically contains degenerative neutrophils and bacteria. Occasionally pustules are difficult to find, but the material under a moist crust

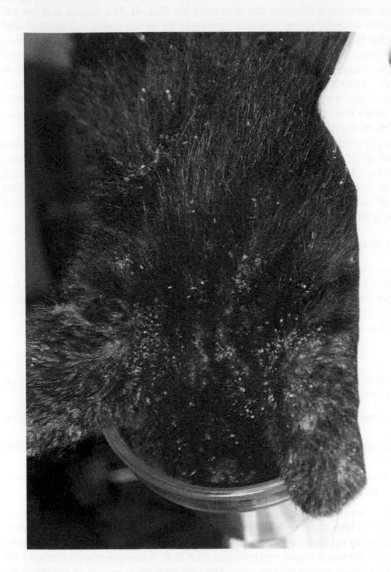

Fig. 2. Scaling of head and ears in a cat with pemphigus foliaceus.

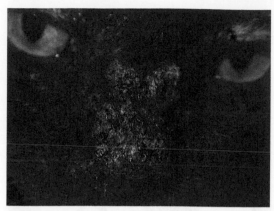

Fig. 3. Symmetric crusting of the dorsal muzzle of cat with pemphigus foliaceus.

can provide very similar if not identical information as a pustule. Superficial pustular dermatophytosis is caused by *Trichophyton* spp. This dermatophyte does not fluoresce with a Wood's lamp. It can produce similar cytologic and histopathologic results. If there is a suspicion of this dermatophyte infection, both hair and crust should be submitted for culture to a laboratory. Typically, this species of dermatophyte can take 3 to 4 weeks to grow out and identify on culture. On biopsy, a periodic acid-Schiff stain can be used to screen for the organism as well.[14]

The histopathology of appropriate lesions can provide the definitive diagnosis of feline PF. Select an intact pustule if possible. Again, if no pustule is found, crusts, especially newer moist crusts, can often provide a definitive diagnosis because new pustules can be forming beneath crusts.[2] If the crust becomes separated from the underlying dermis/epidermis, include it in the formalin and make a note of it to the pathologists so they can include the wayward crust in their sample preparation.

HISTOPATHOLOGIC FINDINGS

The epidermis is mild to severely hyperplastic, mostly owing to acanthosis with a smaller number of samples also having hypergranulosis. The hyperplasia is

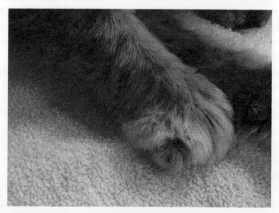

Fig. 4. Paws seem to be dirty, but that is due to crust forming around nails and base of paw pads.

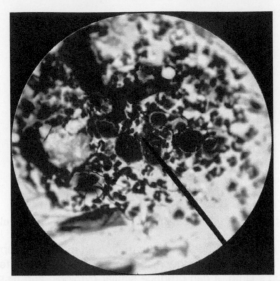

Fig. 5. View through a microscope at 100×; note the mature neutrophils and larger, round, nucleated, bluish-stained acantholytic cells around the tip of the pointer.

predominantly due to orthokeratotic hyperkeratosis, but focal parakeratosis can be noted.[2,3] The dermis shows a mild to severe perivascular to interstitial infiltrate.[2,3] Although the infiltrate is primarily neutrophils, in a large retrospective study 94% of the samples also showed mast cells and they were the predominant cell type in 20% of the samples.[2] Eosinophils were also commonly found, but they were never the predominant cell type.[2] Other cell types reported were lymphocytes and plasma cells.[3,9] In the larger retrospective study, pustules were most commonly located within the stratum corneum (corneal) or both in the corneal and subcorneal layers and the smallest percentage at the level of the stratum spinosum or granulosum (subcorneal). In a little more than one-half of the samples, "rafts" of acantholytic cells, that is, several or more acantholytic cells grouped together, were found and slightly fewer than one-quarter of the samples acantholytic cells were found clinging to the roof of the pustules.[2] Pustules can be seen developing within hair follicles.[2,3,9] Besides acantholytic cells, pustules contain primarily neutrophils and sometimes eosinophils.[2,3,9] When paw pads are biopsied pustules are often preserved by the overlying thick keratin of the footpad.[9] Similar histopathologic findings were reported by Jordan and colleagues,[7] except for 8 cats whose samples showed changes suggestive of a vasculopathy.

The histopathology of drug-related/triggered PF should be the same as naturally occurring PF.[9] One concern when performing biopsies on an animal with suspected autoimmune disorders is the possible effect of concurrent steroid use. In a retrospective study by Preziosi and colleagues,[2] 17 of 57 cats were on steroids at the time of biopsy. It was found that the proportion of diagnostic samples was higher in cats not on steroids at the time of biopsy than the ones on some sort of corticosteroid. However, there was no difference in the number of acantholytic cells or type of dermal infiltrate in the diagnostic samples (see **Box 1** for tips on biopsy).

Immunologic studies are not routinely performed on cats.[14] Intercellular IgG was found in 4 of 8 cats with PF in both blood samples and 1 of 2 samples in the other 4 cats.[3] However, it is clear from research in dogs that intercellular IgG can also be found in the blood of dogs with dermatoses other than PF.[5]

Box 1
Biopsy tips for feline pemphigus foliaceus

1. Discontinue steroids for a week if possible.

2. Treat pyoderma if present for at least 2 weeks.

3. Select representative lesions, pustules if possible, moist crusts are second choice, affected footpads can be great sites.

4. Do not prep the site. If hair is in the way gently clip hair with scissors.

5. Use a punch slightly bigger than the lesion and push and twist firmly so that you pop through without sawing back and forth.

6. Gently lift the skin sample up without squeezing the tissue at all.

7. If the crust falls off despite your best efforts, pick it up and place it the formalin as well.

8. Aim for at least 2 to 4 good samples.

THERAPY

In the past, therapy for feline patients with PF usually depended on prednisone using doses of 2 to 3 mg/kg/d to induce remission over the course of at least 2 weeks and then a gradual taper.[3,4,13] Sometimes, maintaining disease remission necessitated prednisone dosed at 2 mg/kg every other day, additional therapy with chlorambucil, gold salts, or azathioprine, or the cat was switched to other steroids such as dexamethasone or triamcinolone. Many of these drugs caused problems. In a small study of 5 cats, azathioprine was found to cause profound neutropenia, a few cats also had thrombocytopenia, and 1 cat was euthanized owing to a severe respiratory infection.[15] Gold salts are now difficult to find and they can cause thrombocytopenia, toxic epidermal necrosis, stomatitis, proteinuria, sterile abscesses at the injection sites, and rarely hepatic necrosis can also occur. Chlorambucil is a popular addition because it is straightforward to dose. It is an alkylating agent that targets the purine base guanine in DNA causing incompatible cross-linking of the nucleic acid chain, which eventually leads to genetic miscoding and cell death. Anorexia and myelosuppression have been reported.[16] In a study of 24 cats, chlorambucil and prednisone were used to treat PF. Improvement took as long as 4 to 8 weeks in some patients, at which point chlorambucil was decreased to every other day dosing as the prednisone dose was decreased. Most cats were weaned off chlorambucil, but were still on prednisone every other day.[16] Although prednisone alone worked at higher doses for some cats, many cats had to be switched to other drugs or have a second drug added if the dose of prednisone was to be reduced.

In a retrospective study that compared the success of treatment based on the drugs used, it was clear that triamcinolone was a far more successful treatment for feline PF than prednisone, prednisone plus chlorambucil, or dexamethasone.[2] The reason for prednisone being a less effective steroid in many cats became apparent with a study that looked at the pharmacokinetics of prednisone versus prednisolone in 6 cats. It was determined that the maximum serum concentration of oral prednisolone was significantly greater than that of oral prednisone. The authors theorized that there may be less gastrointestinal absorption or less conversion in the liver to the active metabolite, prednisolone.[17] A retrospective study looked at 37 cats that received prednisolone as a monotherapy for PF using an induction dose of 2 mg/kg/d. Complete remission was achieved in 97% of the cats within 8 weeks using this dose. The median maintenance dose was 1.2 mg/kg/wk. In 14% of cats, the medication was eventually discontinued. Adverse effects were uncommon.[18]

The most recent addition to therapy for feline PF is cyclosporine (CsA). CsA is a lipophilic cyclicpolypeptide metabolite of the fungus *Beauveria nivea*. The metabolite is a calcineurin inhibitor preventing transcription of T-cell cytokines such as interleukin-2 that controls T-cell activation and proliferation.[19,20] Besides inhibiting cell-mediated immunity, it has some effect on humoral immunity as well as effects on keratinocytes, mast cells, eosinophils, and epidermal Langerhans cells.[19,20] A study compared 6 cats with PF receiving prednisolone and CsA with 6 that were treated with prednisolone and chlorambucil. All cats in the CsA group responded and eventually were weaned off of prednisolone. Four cats had a good response in the other group, but 3 of those were switched to dexamethasone for long-term use.[12] In the most recent retrospective study, 33 cats went into complete remission and of those 22 were on some type of corticosteroid and 11 were on a corticosteroid with the addition of Cs , chlorambucil, or gold salts. Of the 33 cats, 19 had a relapse at some point when the drug doses were tapered or when an attempt was made to discontinue the drugs. Only 1 cat with a suspected thyroid carcinoma had a spontaneous remission. All the other cats had to stay on medication for life.[7] For cats that experience side effects from steroids or that cannot take steroids, CsA may provide an alternative treatment (**Table 1** provides a summary of recommended therapies).

Once a cat has achieved remission, it is often a difficult decision for both veterinarian and owner to decide how fast to taper the medication. Typically, the owner would like their cat off medication as soon as possible for many reasons and the veterinarian would like their patient to remain in remission. Cats being cats, what a clinician and owner want may not be what they get. The author has come to rely on melt-away prednisolone tablets or flavored liquid triamcinolone as the first therapeutic option using the induction doses listed in **Table 1**. Using prednisolone as an example: dosing for a typical 10- to 12-pound cat translate to about 5 mg of prednisolone twice daily (~2 mg/kg/d), usually for 3 weeks, sometimes longer before the crusts dry up and start to fall off. When that happens, a taper is started. This strategy includes a recheck in 3 weeks to determine if the reduction is appropriate, not the owner's assessment. The first reduction is to 7.5 mg/d and if they are still doing well after 2 weeks, the dose is reduced again to 5 mg/d for another 2 weeks. Then, an attempt is made to taper to 5 mg every other day or 2.5 mg/d with an eventual goal of 2.5 mg every other day or 5 mg 2 to 3 times weekly. If the initial period of improvement took longer, say 4 to 6 weeks for all crusting to resolve, the author will taper over a slightly longer period of time. If improvement is really slow, the author may add CsA (Atopica) early on. The author tends not to use chlorambucil much because repeat complete blood

Table 1
Treatment options for feline pemphigus foliaceus

Drug Name	Induction Dose (mg/kg/d)	Most Common Side Effects	Maintenance Dose (mg/kg)
Prednisolone	2	PU/PD, diabetes	1.2–5.0 q wk
Triamcinolone	0.6–2.0	PU/PD, diabetes	0.6–1.0 q 48 h to q 1 wk
Dexamethasone	0.13–0.2	PU/PD, diabetes	—
Atopica	5–6	V/D, anorexia, gingival hyperplasia	5 q 48–72 h
Chlorambucil	0.15–0.20	Anorexia, vomiting	0.15 q 48–72 h
Chlorambucil	0.38 q 48 h	Anorexia, vomiting	0.15–0.20 q 48–72 h

Abbreviations: D, diarrhea; PU, polyuria; PD, polydipsia; V, vomiting.
Data from Refs.[2,12,16,18]

counts and serum biochemical values will need to be evaluated more often, which cats may not appreciate. Other dermatologists may favor other drugs or other tapering schemes. This example is meant to provide guidance.

DISCUSSION

When a cat is presented with a rapid onset of a mostly symmetric crusting disorder that affects the head and feet, PF should be high on the differential list. Taking samples for cytology from pustules and crusts in the examination room to look for neutrophils, bacteria, or acantholytic cells and trichograms to evaluate for fungal arthrospores or to help decide if you want to submit a fungal culture are all necessary tests to help hone your differential list. From there, a decision can be made if there is enough evidence to biopsy, and make the proper lesion selection. Once a diagnosis of feline PF is made, treatment is likely to center on the use of steroids, either prednisolone or triamcinolone, with drugs such as CsA and chlorambucil used as adjunctive or replacement therapy when needed. Many cats will require therapy for the long term and possibly low doses of medication for life, but can live with a good quality of life.

REFERENCES

1. Griffin CE, Campbell KL, Miller WH. Autoimmune and immune-mediated dermatoses. In: Muller & Kirk's small animal dermatology. 7th edition. Philadelphia: WB Saunders Co.; 2013. p. 438–48.
2. Preziosi DE, Goldschmidt MH, Greek JS, et al. Feline pemphigus foliaceus: a retrospective analysis of 57 cases. Vet Dermatol 2003;14:313–21.
3. Canciolo PL, Nesbitt GH, Hurvitz AI. Pemphigus foliaceus in eight cats and results of induction therapy using azathioprine. J Amer An Hosp Assoc 1984;20:571–7.
4. Manning TO, Scott DW, Smith CA, et al. Pemphigus diseases in the feline: seven case reports and discussion. J Amer An Hosp Assoc 1982;18:433–43.
5. Olivry T, Chan LS. Autoimmune blistering dermatoses in domestic animals. Clin Dermatol 2001;19:750–60.
6. Lambacher B, Schoiswohl J, Brunthaler R, et al. Successful treatment of pemphigus foliaceus in a Berrichon du Cher ram with methylprednisolone acetate. Vet Dermatol 2017;28:499–502.
7. Jordan TJM, Affolter VK, et al. Clinicopathological findings and clinical outcomes in 49 cases of feline pemphigus foliaceus examined in northern California, USA (1987-2017). Abstract from N Amer Vet Derm Forum May 2018.
8. Brenner S, Bialy-Golan A, Ruocco V. Drug induced pemphigus. Clin Dermatol 1998;16:393–7.
9. Gross TL, Ihrke PJ, Walder EJ. Diseases of the epidermis. In: Skin diseases of the dog and cat. clinical and histopathologic diagnosis. 2nd edition. IA): Blackwell Science; 2005. p. 14–8.
10. McEwan NA, McNeil PE, Kirkham D, et al. Drug eruption in a cat resembling pemphigus foliaceus. J Sm An Prac 1987;28:713–20.
11. Mason KV, Day MJ. A pemphigus foliaceus-like eruption associated with the use of ampicillin in a cat. Aust Vet J 1987;64:223–4.
12. Irwin KE, Beale KM, Fadok VA. Use of modified ciclosporin in the management of feline pemphigus foliaceus: a retrospective analysis. Vet Dermatol 2012;23:403–9.
13. Griffin CE. Recognizing and treating pemphigus foliaceus in cats. Vet Med 1991;86:513–6.

14. Tater KC, Olivry T. Canine and feline pemphigus foliaceus: improving your chances of a successful outcome. Available at: http://www.dvm360.com. Accessed February 10, 2018.
15. Beale KM, Altman D, Clemmons RR, et al. Systemic toxicosis associated with azathioprine administration in domestic cats. Am J Vet Res 1992;53:1236–40.
16. Rhoades KH, Sholberg N. Chorambucil: effective therapeutic options for the treatment of feline immune-mediated dermatoses. Fel Prac 1992;20:5–8.
17. Graham-Mize CA, Rosser EJ. Bioavailability and activity of prednisone and prednisolone in the feline patient. Vet Dermatol 2004;15:10.
18. Simpson DL, Burton GC. Use of prednisolone as monotherapy in the treatment of feline pemphigus foliaceus: a retrospective study of 37 cats. Vet Dermatol 2013; 24:598–601.
19. Madan V, Griffiths CEM. Systemic ciclosporin and tacrolimus in dermatology. Dermatol Ther 2007;20:239–50.
20. Robson D. Review of the properties and mechanisms of action of cyclosporine with an emphasis on dermatological therapy in dogs, cats and people. Vet Rec 2003;152:768–72.

Diagnosis and Treatment of Canine Acral Lick Dermatitis

Amy K. Shumaker, DVM

KEYWORDS

- Acral lick dermatitis • Obsessive-compulsive disorder • Dog

KEY POINTS

- Acral lick dermatitis is a common, frustrating disease characterized by incessant licking behavior resulting in ulcerative, firm plaques.
- The disease is caused by underlying primary triggers (allergic disorders, orthopedic or neurologic disorders, infectious disease, parasitic diseases, neoplasia, or a psychogenic disorder).
- Secondary infections commonly complicate the disorder and need to be appropriately addressed.
- A behavioral component (either primary or contributory) may need to be treated by behavioral modification and potentially psychopharmacologic drug interventions.

INTRODUCTION

Acral lick dermatitis (ALD), also referred to as acral lick granuloma or acral pruritic nodule, is a common disease in dogs, occurring in 2.9% of 559 dermatologic cases in one study.[1] Caused by incessant licking behavior, this can be a frustrating disorder, having an impact on the quality of life of the patient as well as the owners. ALD has been described in cattle, various zoo and exotic animal species, as well as humans.[2–5] As common as this disorder is, there has been little published on the diagnosis and treatment of this frustrating disease. Most publications have focused on behavioral modification or behavior-modifying drugs for treatment. Although many cases may have a psychogenic component that ultimately plays a role later in the disease process, an underlying primary organic disease is often the inciting trigger, with an allergic disorder being the leading causative factor suspected by most dermatologists. In either case, secondary bacterial infections often are associated with ALD[6] and continue to perpetuate the pruritus and licking behavior. Successful management of ALD requires an understanding of the multifactorial cause of this condition.

Disclosure: Nothing to disclose.
VCA South Shore Animal Hospital, 595 Columbian Street, South Weymouth, MA 02190, USA
E-mail address: akshumaker@yahoo.com

Vet Clin Small Anim 49 (2019) 105–123
https://doi.org/10.1016/j.cvsm.2018.08.010
0195-5616/19/© 2018 Elsevier Inc. All rights reserved.

PRESENTATION

ALD can affect dogs of any age, and there are conflicting reports regarding typical age of onset, with one study of 31 dogs having an age range of 1 to 12 years and median age of onset of 4 years.[6] Large breeds tend to be more affected, with the Doberman pinscher, Great Dane, Labrador retriever, golden retriever, German shepherd, boxer, Weimaraner, and Irish setter as reported predisposed dog breeds.[7,8] Lesions appear as well-circumscribed, raised, alopecic, indurated, often erosive to ulcerative plaques on the cranial distal extremities but have been reported at other sites. Shumaker and colleagues,[6] noted a trend toward a female predisposition, although not statistically significant, which was found to be in contrast with other reports in which no predilection or a male sex predilection was reported. When only a unilateral lesion was present, the cranial left carpal region was predominantly affected.

PATHOGENESIS

The creation of an acral lick lesion is often multifactorial, with the lesion evolving over time. Frequent licking at an affected site initially may result in a haired lesion with underlying erythema, scaling, and crusting, progressing to alopecia and erosion. Exposure of the deeper layers of the epidermis, dermis, and the sensory nerve fibers elicits pruritus and perpetuates the itch-lick cycle. With chronicity, marked dermal fibrosis and epidermal hyperplasia develop, creating the plaque appearance of the lesion. Folliculitis and furunculosis are often present and are a consequence of both the licking behavior (hairs forced deep into the lesion) and secondary infection. In many cases, hidradenitis and epitrichial gland dilatation and rupture may be present.[6] The presence of folliculitis, furunculosis, free keratin, and ruptured glandular secretions create foreign body reactions, additionally perpetuating the cycle.

As in ear disease, ALD can be viewed as having primary and perpetuating factors. The primary factors are the initiating cause for the development of the ALD, with the perpetuating factors being a continuing driving force to lick the affected areas, even if the primary factor is transient, such as an allergic flare. Primary organic factors include allergic disorders (atopic disease, cutaneous adverse food reaction, flea allergic dermatitis); bacterial or fungal disease (including dermatophytosis), parasitic disorders (demodicosis, scabies), previous trauma, joint disease, foreign body, neoplasia, neuropathy, or hormonal disorders. Primary psychogenic disorders include stereotypic or obsessive-compulsive disorder (OCD), anxiety, boredom, attention seeking, or stress. Perpetuating factors include secondary bacterial infections, keratin foreign bodies as a result of licking and furunculosis, bony changes such as osteomyelitis or periostitis, and development of a secondary compulsive disorder/learned behavior.

DIAGNOSTIC WORK-UP

As with most dermatologic diseases, a thorough history is necessary to best elucidate which primary factor may be involved in triggering the licking behavior and to tailor the work-up and treatment. **Box 1** reviews questions to consider when evaluating patients with ALD to better direct the diagnostic work-up and perhaps shorten the list of possible primary triggers.

A thorough dermatologic examination may reveal evidence of other areas of the body being affected, suggesting an allergic disorder. A frequently missed area on examination often involved in allergic disorders is the ventral interdigital aspects of paws. This region can be erythemic even in cases in which clients do not note obvious paw

---

Box 1
Historical questions to review with owners in cases of acral lick dermatitis

Allergic:
    Is the dog showing any signs of pruritus elsewhere (licking/chewing/rubbing/scratching)?
    Any history of past or current skin infections or any history of otitis?
    Any history of gastrointestinal disease that may support a food allergy?
    Any seasonality to symptoms or seasonal exacerbations noted if the lesions are persistent for
    a year or more?

Orthopedic/neurologic:
    Any history of trauma to the affected leg?
    Any indication of joint pain (eg, limping)?

Behavioral:
    Are there any other concurrent behavioral symptoms (eg, separation anxiety, noise phobia,
    tail chasing) that would support a primary compulsive disorder/OCD behavior?
    Have there been any major changes to the dog's environment (recent move, new people/
    babies/pet introduced into the house)?
    Any recent deaths (family member or companion to the dog)?
    How much exercise (walk, play) and socialization does the dog receive? Ask extent of time.
    Is the dog kept indoors or outdoors?
    How long is the dog left alone during the day?
    Is the dog kept confined (crate, kennel/run)?
    Are there other animals in the home? What are the relationships with the other animals?
    What sort of toys are available and are they used by the dog?

---

licking. Ears should also be evaluated as a part of every dermatologic examination, with disease occasionally noted in apparently asymptomatic dogs.

An orthopedic examination should be performed to evaluate for any indication of underlying joint disease. If the lesion overlies a joint, placing that joint through flexion/extension may unveil the presence of crepitus or result in elicitable pain. The opposite joint should be evaluated for comparison. Radiographs can be helpful in evaluating for presence of arthritis or other signs of trauma. Osteomyelitis or periostitis may be detected on radiographs; presence of these changes can potentially be a poor prognostic indicator for satisfactory resolution.[8]

In cases showing possible neurologic abnormalities or that have a past history of trauma (eg, hit by car), a neurologic examination and work-up should be performed. Needle electromyography (EMG) and nerve conduction velocity studies may be useful in identifying abnormalities in nerve conduction. In one study evaluating tricyclic antidepressants for treatment of ALD in which EMG studies were being performed as part of the work-up, 9 of 16 dogs (56%) had EMG abnormalities involving the same side (or sides if bilateral) of the lesion.[9] Several of the dogs in this study did have prior history of trauma. Although not practical or likely to yield useful information in most cases, in those cases with a history of trauma, an EMG study may be useful in identifying an underlying nerve root lesion or neuropathy.

Laboratory work (complete blood count, biochemistry, thyroid profile, urinalysis) can be helpful in ruling out any endocrinopathies that may be an underlying trigger. Skin scrapings and hair plucks should be performed to evaluate for presence of mites. Hair samples from within the lesion and the periphery can be obtained for culture on dermatophyte test medium to evaluate for presence of dermatophytes. The Mackenzie toothbrush technique can also be used to acquire some scale, crust, and hairs from the lesion for plating.[10] Dermatophyte cultures should be allowed to grow for 21 days with daily monitoring of the plate for growth and color change of the medium.

Any suspicious colonies should be evaluated microscopically to identify macroconidia and not based solely on color change because saprophytic fungal organisms can also change color on the media plates, although this color change usually occurs after growth. The plate can also be submitted to a reference laboratory for identification for clinicians who are unsure or uncomfortable about identifying dermatophytes microscopically. Alternatively, hair and scale samples can be submitted to IDEXX for a Dermatophyte RealPCR test, which tests for the presence of DNA of the more common dermatophyte species, with results typically available within 3 days of submission.

Cytology should be performed to evaluate for the presence of secondary infection. Ideally, the lesion should be squeezed to express fluid from the deeper tissue. Cytology is not only useful in helping to identify infection but can aid in monitoring response to treatment at subsequent visits. Presence or absence of infectious organisms and inflammatory cells should be recorded for sequential comparisons. However, if there is poor response to empirical antibiotic therapy based on cytologic findings, culture should be performed because cytology was found to correlate poorly with superficial and deep tissue culture results in a prior study.[6] Bacterial cultures are useful in guiding decisions on antimicrobial therapy. However, in the case of ALD lesions, tissue culture by biopsy should be submitted as opposed to a swab sample from the surface because there was poor correlation between superficial and deep tissue isolates, with only 36% agreement between the two.[6] A nonulcerated site should be selected, sterilely prepped to remove any surface contaminants, and tissue obtained using a 6-mm punch biopsy. The tissue is then submitted in either a Port-A-Cul tube or a sterile tube containing a small amount of sterile, nonbacteriostatic saline for transfer. The tissue is then macerated at the reference laboratory for culture.

Neoplasia can be an underlying trigger for ALD or chronic licking, and cytologic or histopathologic evaluation can help to differentiate these lesions. Fine-needle aspiration may be helpful in aiding in diagnosis of neoplasia, but it does not necessarily rule it out. Cytology may reveal the presence of inflammatory cells, fibrocytes, and possibly infectious organisms, supporting a diagnosis of ALD. Biopsy with histopathology can differentiate between a possible neoplastic process or underlying fungal disease, or can further support a diagnosis of ALD. Typical histopathologic findings are described in **Box 2**, with several of these histopathologic features highlighted in **Fig. 1**.

Box 2
Common histopathologic findings in acral lick dermatitis

- Moderate to marked, frequently papillated acanthosis
- Erosion or ulceration with exudation
- Occasional neutrophilic serocellular crusts
- Hyperkeratosis
- Dermal fibrosis in a vertical streaking pattern
- Thickened and elongated follicles
- Dermal infiltrate of lymphocytes, neutrophils, macrophages, and plasma cells in a perivascular, perifollicular, or diffuse pattern
- Dilatation, hypertrophy of epitrichial glands, often with retained secretions
- Perihidradenitis and hidradenitis with occasional gland rupture
- Folliculitis and furunculosis

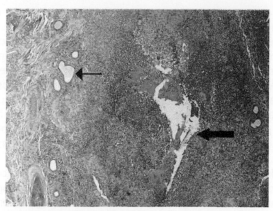

Fig. 1. Common histopathologic features of an acral lick granuloma, including marked lymphoplasmacytic inflammation, a ruptured hair follicle with a free hair (*large arrow*), hidradenitis, and dilated epitrichial glands with retained secretions (*small arrow*) (H&E, original magnification ×4).

As previously mentioned, ALD can manifest as a stereotypic or obsessive-compulsive disorder as the primary underlying trigger. ALD has been proposed to serve as an animal analog for human OCD.[11–14] In dogs, compulsive disorders are defined as repetitive behaviors occurring out of context and are not easily interrupted or deterred by normal stimuli.[15] A thorough history, as outlined in **Box 1**, is critical when trying to elucidate whether a psychogenic component is driving the licking in ALD. It has been estimated that up to 70% of dogs with ALD may have other anxiety-related conditions[16]; therefore, a comorbid anxiety disorder with lack of concurrent allergic or orthopedic symptoms would lend support to a psychogenic disorder. In an evaluation of 20 dogs presenting with ALD with psychogenic triggers, 70% were confined to small areas, 64% were not permitted to stay inside the house, none of the owners played with their dogs on a routine basis, 70% were never taken for walks, all of the owners considered their dogs to have an anxious disposition, and 65% had a nonmedical triggering component (eg, death of a canine companion) identified.[17] Thus, these findings stress the importance of determining whether the dog is environmentally deprived, undergoing stress or conflict, or displaying any other comorbid anxiety disorders via a detailed, investigative history.

TREATMENT

Successful treatment and prevention of recurrence of ALD is contingent on addressing the primary and perpetuating factors: identification and resolution or control of the underlying trigger, treating infection, and breaking the itch-lick cycle. If these 3 factors are not addressed, resolution without recurrence is not likely. It is important to stress to clients that resolution will take time, and frequently different therapies are attempted before the right one (or combination) is found.

Breaking the Itch-Lick Cycle

Preventing access to the acral lick site is another essential step in resolution. Healing is unlikely to occur if the dog is permitted to continue to lick the site even if the primary factor and underlying infection are appropriately addressed. Physical restraint needs to be tailored to the dog and the owner. Elizabethan collars are often effective, but many dogs can still access the lesion around these collars and many clients find them cumbersome and are reluctant to maintain them on their dog for the extended period of time needed for resolution of the lesion. BiteNot collars may be effective in preventing access to some lesions and are much more acceptable to the dog and owners, but many dogs can still get around to access the lesion. Socks and booties are effective barriers for some dogs, but others are adept at removing them. A more durable wrap that can be custom made for the dog based on measurements can be found on www.dogleggs.com. Often selection of a means of physical restraint may take trial and error. Once the lesion is resolved, the selected form of physical restraint can be removed for short periods initially while supervising the dog, slowly increasing the time without the restraint if no licking is observed.

Topicals can also be effective at deterring some of the licking behavior. Certain sprays, such as bitter apple, may be noxious enough to some dogs. A mixture of HEET with bitter apple in a 1:2 ratio applied on or around the granuloma up to 3 times daily has been used with success in others.[18] HEET is a liniment containing capsaicin as one of its active ingredients. Capsaicin, a chili pepper extract, contains analgesic properties and has been shown to be effective in reducing neuropathic pain[19,20] as well as neuropathic pruritus[21] and pruritus[22] in humans. Capsaicin was observed by owners to reduce pruritus in affected dogs, but no significant improvement was noted by investigators; further studies were recommended by the investigators.[23]

Oral steroids and topical steroids can also be helpful at reducing the inflammation and pruritus associated with these lesions. Synotic (fluocinolone with dimethyl sulfoxide [DMSO]) can be an especially effective topical agent because the DMSO aids in increasing the penetration of the fluocinolone through the thickened tissue. Other products, such as Tresaderm and Otomax, may also be effective topicals because they contain a combination of steroid and antibiotics, which may help further treat secondary infection, although this should not replace systemic antibiotic therapy. Intralesional injectable steroids are generally discouraged because of the likelihood of concurrent infection, but they may be considered once infection has been adequately addressed.

Infection

Because most ALD lesions are secondarily infected, systemic antimicrobial therapy is vital. Prolonged courses of 6 to 8 weeks or longer (occasionally several months) may be required to resolve infections. If empiric treatment is initially selected (eg, cephalosporins) with poor response despite appropriate dose and treatment course, then therapy should be selected based on culture (ideally tissue culture) as previously discussed.

Allergic Disorders

The primary trigger in most cases is likely an underlying allergy. An elimination diet trial with a commercial prescription or home-cooked diet should be performed. In the past, elimination diet trials are performed from 6 to 12 weeks; however, the disease should be completely resolved before challenging the diet to best ascertain whether a food allergy is driving the behavior. Too often secondary infections or perpetuating factors are not appropriately treated/resolved or addressed during an elimination diet trial, potentially misleading the veterinarian into ruling out a food allergy as the primary disease. With chronic lesions, resolution may take several months between treating the infection with an appropriate course of antibiotics, and inflammation with oral and/or topical steroids, as well as breaking the itch-lick cycle, before a dietary challenge can be instituted. If a food allergy has been ruled out or is not suspected based on history (seasonal exacerbations), then work-up and treatment of environmental allergies is warranted. Treatment options include allergen testing and immunotherapy (see Ralf S. Mueller's article, Update on Allergen Immunotherapy, in this issue), Apoquel (oclacitinib), or Atopica (cyclosporine). Allergen-specific immunotherapy based on testing (intradermal or serology) may be an effective means of controlling underlying atopic dermatitis and should be considered as a viable means of treatment; however, this therapy takes time to show benefit (several months to a year), so this should be used as a long-term treatment and adjunctive therapies may be needed until benefit is noted. Institution of therapy with oclacitinib or cyclosporine should be performed after infections have been appropriately addressed. Oral steroids could be a consideration for long-term therapy, but, because of potential adverse side effects, the other therapies should be attempted before resorting to this option, and owners should be appropriately educated regarding long-term side effects.

Orthopedic

If an underlying orthopedic issue is discovered, appropriate measures should be taken to reduce pain (eg, with nonsteroidal antiinflammatory drugs) or to correct the underlying problem.

Laser Ablation

Lasers are becoming increasingly used in veterinary medicine. The CO_2 laser is an efficient instrument at incising tissue and providing hemostasis as well as effectively ablating proliferative tissue or tumors. CO_2 lasers have many advantages, including sealing small blood vessels less than 0.5 mm, sealing lymph vessels and nerve endings, and vaporizing tissue (including tumor cells) and bacteria, thus sterilizing the treated area.[24] In addition, there is less postoperative pain with CO_2 lasers compared with traditional surgery; however, laser surgery is painful at the time of procedure, and patients need general or local anesthesia depending on the size, location, and type of lesion.

For ALD, laser ablation should be considered as a treatment option once potential underlying triggers have been addressed, infections resolved, and if the lesion is persisting. Laser ablation should not be considered a first-line therapy without addressing infection and triggers because the lesion will likely recur. In addition to the benefits of laser ablation mentioned earlier, in the case of ALD lesions, it can also be useful for removal of deep pyogranulomatous tracts[25] as well as sealing nerve endings, potentially decreasing some of the sensory nerve sensation triggering the pruritus. Note that the CO_2 laser only penetrates to a depth of about 0.3 mm; therefore, when ablating a large ALD lesion, the procedure may need to be staged because ablation to a satisfactory depth takes time. Alternatively, the lesion can first be debulked with the laser, then the remaining tissue ablated.[26]

Successful laser surgery requires skill, knowledge of the physics of laser, and understanding laser safety. There are often workshops provided at continuing education meetings. In addition, there are online courses, including those provided by the American Laser Study Club or the American Institute of Medical Laser Applications.

Surgery

Traditional surgical excision may be difficult and have complications. Because most lesions overlie flexural regions, concern for dehiscence postoperatively from joint motion exists. In addition, the size of the lesion often precludes surgical excision because wound closure may not be possible because of limitations of location. For those lesions that are small enough for surgical excision, there is still concern that the licking behavior may persist postoperatively if the underlying trigger has not been appropriately addressed before surgical intervention.

Cryosurgery

Cryosurgery, also known as cryotherapy, has also been reported as a treatment option, although to the author's knowledge there are no published reports on use with ALD, and it has not been used as a treatment of ALD by this author. A cryogen, typically liquid nitrogen, is used to cool tissue to subzero temperatures, inducing tissue damage by 2 different mechanisms.[27] First, freezing of the tissue induces tissue ischemia by damaging blood vessels and capillaries within the target zone, resulting in ischemic necrosis. Second, additional cellular damage is achieved by formation of ice crystals, inducing osmotic cell injury and cellular membrane disruption. Ice crystals form between the cells as the tissue is cooled, creating an osmotic gradient, pulling water out of the cells. With continued cooling, crystals form within the cell, possibly resulting in cellular rupture. Crystals outside the cells melt as the tissue thaws, creating an osmotic gradient, pulling water back into the cell, resulting in swelling and rupturing of the cell. Two to 3 freeze-thaw cycles are typically used to treat cutaneous or subcutaneous tumors in veterinary medicine because the amount of tissue damage increases with each freeze-thaw cycle.[28]

Cryosurgery holds appeal as a treatment option for many lesions because it only requires local anesthesia for most lesions. However, in anxious animals or those with painful lesions, such as with ALD, light sedation may be required. In addition, the size and thickness of the lesion may be a limiting factor because the treated tissue can often only be effectively cooled to a certain depth. Therefore, large, thickened ALD lesions are likely to need to be retreated following adequate healing from the prior treatment. Keratin is a poor conductor and could affect the depth of freeze[27]; therefore, if the ALD lesion being treated is hyperkeratotic, debulking before performing cryosurgery may improve response to treatment.

Radiation Therapy

Radiation therapy has been used as a treatment of ALD, and it is suspected that the X-ray irradiation destroys nerve endings in the affected area, breaking the itch-lick cycle. Treatment with radiation therapy has been shown to have some satisfactory results. In one study, it was reported that about 50% of dogs with acropruritic granulomas healed without recurrence; however, follow-up time was not provided.[29] In another study, 11 of 13 cases had good results; however, there was recurrence at the site in 5 dogs with new lesions developing at other sites in 3 dogs.[30] Healing was satisfactory in most dogs. The frequency of recurrence or development of new lesions that occurred in this study emphasizes the necessity of identifying and addressing underlying triggers before undertaking certain treatment modalities.

Acupuncture

Acupuncture involves insertion of needles along meridians into specific acupoints. A form of energy, qi, is theorized to travel along these meridians. Placement of needles and subsequent stimulation can alter qi. It has been suggested that pruritus may be alleviated by acupuncture along a similar neural pathway to that of pain.[31] Human studies suggest that acupuncture can be effective at reducing pruritus.[32,33] Acupuncture involves stimulation of A delta nerve fibers. The stimulated interneurons are activated in the dorsal horn of the spinal cord, producing encephalons, and inhibiting C-fiber activity in the dorsal horn. Segmental acupuncture may have an effect by needling close to the area where C-fiber pain originates and manipulating areas supplied by the same segment of the spinal cord.[31] Pruritus and pain are both transmitted along C fibers; however, it is unclear whether they travel along the same or different fibers, and it is currently thought that pruritus travels along different C fibers.[34]

It is thought that ALD is an obstruction of the flow of energy, or qi, along the acupuncture channel or meridian underlying the lesion. Acupuncture treatment points selected locally, proximally, and distally to the lesion can facilitate the clearing of the obstruction; however, needles should not be placed directly into the lesion.[31] "Surrounding the dragon" is an acupuncture technique whereby the needles are inserted surrounding the border of the ALD lesion, directed inward. Another study showed resolution of an acral lick lesion present for 3 months after 3 acupuncture treatments with needles placed at 4 points: the fourth, sixth, and eleventh point of the meridian of large intestine (IC-4, IC-6, and IC-11) and the fourth point of the small intestine (IT-6).[35]

Behavioral/Psychogenic

If it is determined that behavior is an underlying primary factor or is contributing as a secondary factor, then behavioral modification and/or psychopharmacologic treatment will be needed. Environment may need to be altered and enriched as to allow more exercise and social interaction of the dog. Exercise and play activity should be encouraged. Because punishment may increase the anxiety and fear often present in dogs with compulsive disorders, this is not a recommended approach to treatment.[15] In addition, punishment (scolding, reprimanding, hitting, physically stopping the dog from licking) may inadvertently reinforce the behavior as attention-seeking behavior. Alternatively, wanted behaviors could be enforced by applying negative punishment by ignoring the unwanted behaviors consistently (walking away when the dog engages in the unwanted behavior; ie, licking).[15]

In addition to behavioral modification, psychopharmacologic interventions may be required. In many cases, therapy is only temporary until the dog responds to behavioral modifications in the environment. Others require long-term drug therapy.

Several studies have shown improvement in dogs placed on selective serotonin reuptake inhibitors (SSRIs) for treatment of ALD.[12-14] Improvement was noted with SSRIs at doses similar to that used to treat humans with OCD, which suggests that, in those dogs with a psychogenic component to their ALD, the serotonin system is likely involved. The dorsal raphe nucleus contains serotonin neurons that provide most of the serotonergic input to forebrain structures involved in complex emotional response regulation to stress.[36] The serotonergic system is involved in numerous diverse processes, including pain perception, aggression, sleep, sexual behavior, hormone secretion, thermoregulation, motor activity, and food intake, although it is not generally involved in self-grooming.[14] However, a study in cats identified a serotonin subsystem within the dorsal raphe that is selectively activated by chewing or grooming. This finding may support a similar system in dogs that becomes inappropriately activated in ALD.[14] The most commonly studied, efficacious, and currently used SSRI for ALD is fluoxetine.[13-15]

Pharmacotherapeutic drugs other than SSRIs have also been shown to be efficacious with various responses for treatment of ALD, indicating that more than 1 neurotransmitter or factors other than serotonin may be involved. Clomipramine, a tricyclic antidepressant (TCA), has been shown to be effective in placebo-controlled studies.[37] TCAs block reuptake of both serotonin and norepinephrine, whereas SSRIs are more specific, blocking only reuptake of serotonin; therefore, SSRIs are generally associated with fewer adverse side effects. Naltrexone, a narcotic antagonist, was shown to improve lesions in 63% of affected dogs in one study, with regression once the treatment was discontinued.[38] The exact mechanism of action of narcotic antagonists for treatment of stereotypical behaviors is unknown; however, narcotic antagonists antagonize the effects of endogenous opioids via binding to opioid receptors.[39] The dopaminergic system has been implicated in stereotypical behaviors, with interaction between this system and endogenous opioids, thus this may explain the improvement in affected dogs treated with naltrexone.

In those dogs showing a psychogenic component as their likely primary trigger, a consult with a veterinary behaviorist may be warranted for development of the best treatment plan between behavioral modifications and pharmacologic interventions.

CASES
Case 1

Figs. 2–4 show successful treatment and resolution of an ALD lesion by laser ablation on the left metacarpal region of an 8-year-old, male, neutered Doberman pinscher that was originally noted shortly after a digit amputation. Treatment with systemic

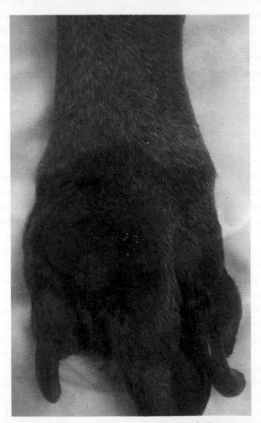

Fig. 2. Alopecic, erythemic, ulcerated, erosive and ulcerated plaque consistent with acral lick granuloma in a Doberman pinscher following digit amputation.

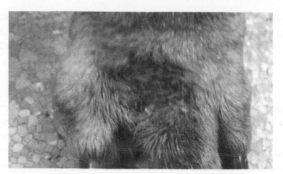

Fig. 3. Two weeks after surgery: reduction is noted in the size of the granuloma with resolution of the thickening of the plaque.

antimicrobial therapies, topical steroids, and systemic behavior-modifying drugs minimally improved the lesion. Physical restraint via E-collar was unsuccessful. Because the suspected trigger was the surgical removal of the digit, drawing attention to the area or possibly triggering pain and initiating the licking behavior, laser ablation was elected because one of the benefits would be sealing the nerve endings in the area, thus relieving any pain that may be triggering licking behavior. At 2 weeks after laser

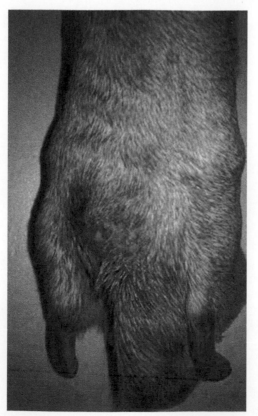

Fig. 4. Six weeks after surgery: almost complete resolution of the lesion with almost complete hair regrowth.

ablation and antimicrobial therapy based on tissue culture (see **Fig. 3**), there was adequate healing from the laser with some hair regrowth. At 6 weeks after the procedure (see **Fig. 4**), almost complete hair regrowth of the original affected site can be appreciated.

Case 2

A 6-year-old, male, intact Doberman pinscher presented for a 9-month history of chronic licking of the left carpal region, resulting in a large, raised, alopecic, indurated plaque with areas of erosion, ulceration, and exudation (**Fig. 5**). The patient did not show any other signs of pruritic behavior and had no history of dermatologic disease before onset of the lesion. He received regular exercise and did not seem to show any other anxiety disorders. When reviewing the history, it was discovered that the licking behavior was first noted shortly after the owner's friend had taken the dog on a strenuous 21-km (13 mile) walk/hike, resulting in some lameness, which had resolved at the time of the dermatology appointment. While performing an orthopedic examination, slight pain appeared to be elicited on flexion of the left carpus compared with the right. Skin scrapings were negative for mites. Cytology from expressed exudate revealed moderate suppurative inflammation with clusters of coccoid bacteria. Sedated radiographs (**Figs. 6** and **7**) of the affected region revealed a jagged lucent line through the

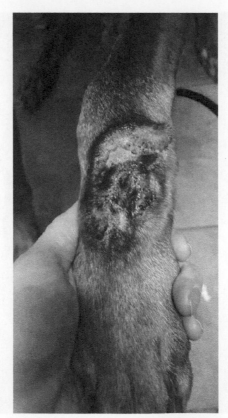

Fig. 5. Large erosive and ulcerated alopecic plaque overlying the left metacarpal/carpal region in a Doberman pinscher.

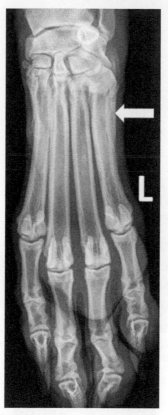

Fig. 6. Radiographs reveal a jagged radiolucent line (*arrow*) through the lateral cortex of metacarpal 5.

lateral cortex of metacarpus 5 with evidence of remodeling, indicating a healing metacarpal fracture. Presence of a rough periosteal margin of metacarpus 3 and 5 was compatible with chronic active osteitis. Soft tissue thickening was appreciated over the dorsal aspect. Based on these findings, it was suspected that underlying orthopedic disease was the primary factor. Cephalexin was instituted empirically based on cytologic findings (owner declined culture). Synotic was recommended to be applied topically until recheck. Carprofen was instituted to address the orthopedic disease.

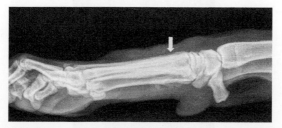

Fig. 7. Soft tissue thickening can be appreciated overlying the carpus and metacarpus. Irregular endosteal changes that indicate osteitis (*arrow*) are present.

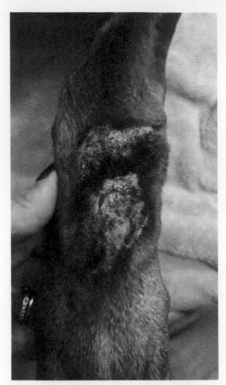

Fig. 8. A decrease in the size of the acral lick granuloma and degree of erosion and ulceration can be appreciated at the week 4 recheck.

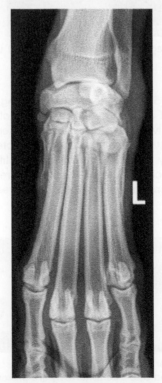

Fig. 9. Progressive healing of the metacarpal fracture can be appreciated.

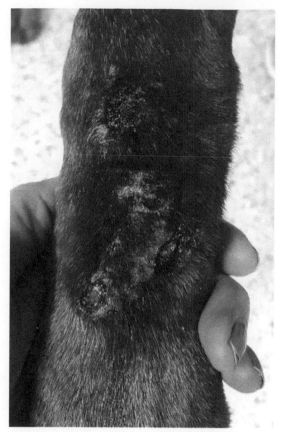

Fig. 10. Continued reduction in the size, thickening, and erosion can be appreciated at the 8-week recheck. Noticeable hair regrowth is present.

Rest was recommended (no heavy exercise, leash walks only) until recheck. A durable leg wrap was recommended because the owner was unable to maintain an Elizabethan collar on the dog. At 4 weeks, the lesion was reduced in size with improved erosion and ulceration (**Fig. 8**). Sedated radiographs (**Fig. 9**) revealed progressive healing of the lesion. The carprofen was discontinued, but cephalexin and Synotic were continued. At the 8-week recheck (**Fig. 10**), continued regression of the lesion was noted with minimal erosion and ulceration and noticeable hair regrowth. The owner was no longer needing to maintain any sort of wrap or other physical restraint to prevent licking of the lesion. Two months later, there was almost complete resolution of the lesion.

Case 3

A 10-year-old female spayed beagle presented for a 4-month history of chronic licking of the left forepaw, resulting in an acral lick granuloma (**Fig. 11**). She had a prior history of nonseasonal recurrent otitis and pedal pruritus with seasonal exacerbations. In the past, oclacitinib seemed to control her pruritus; however, the owner thought that it no longer was controlling the pruritus or the otitis. Before

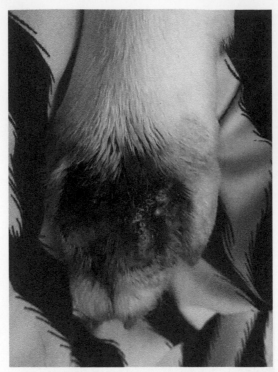

Fig. 11. Thickened, alopecic, erythemic plaque overlying the left dorsal distal metacarpal/digital region.

presentation, she had been on 2-week to 3-week courses of amoxicillin, enrofloxacin, and ketoconazole to treat the acral lick granuloma with no significant improvement. A prescription diet trial with a prescription hydrolyzed protein diet had been started 4 weeks before initial examination. Previous laboratory work performed by the referring veterinarian was unremarkable. Skin scrapings were negative. Cytology from expressible exudate revealed pyogranulomatous inflammation with 1+ intra- and extracellular coccoid bacteria based on 0-4+ scale). The owner declined sedated tissue biopsy for culture but permitted culture from expressible exudate, which isolated methicillin-sensitive *Staphylococcus pseudintermedius*. A 6-week course of cephalexin was recommended (with possible extension based on assessed clinical response at recheck). Synotic was recommended to be applied twice daily for 2 weeks, then once daily for 2 weeks, then every other day until recheck. The owner was instructed to start oral cyclosporine about 2 weeks after starting cephalexin. Because the patient was already in an Elizabethan collar, the owner was instructed to maintain use of the collar until she thought that it could be removed without the patient licking the lesion. The prescription diet trial was recommended to be continued. At the 6-week recheck, almost complete resolution of the acral lick granuloma was noted with almost complete hair regrowth (**Fig. 12**). The owner reported minimal pruritus. The patient no longer needed the Elizabethan collar. The owner was instructed to continue cyclosporine and recommended topicals; the cephalexin course was discontinued.

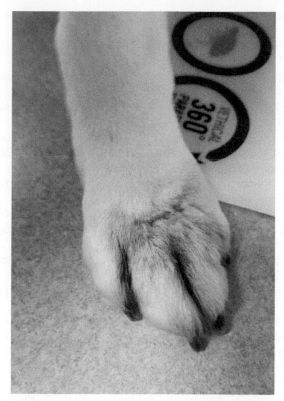

Fig. 12. Virtually complete resolution of the lesion is appreciated after 6 weeks of treatment.

SUMMARY

In the past, it was common to diagnose the inciting trigger of an acral lick lesion as a psychogenic or behavioral disorder. It is now known that this disorder is more complicated, involving numerous potential underlying primary and perpetuating factors, and, as such, merits a thorough diagnostic work-up in order to identify the primary trigger, whether organic, psychogenic, or a combination, and to tailor the appropriate treatment plan. As with many conditions, a multimodal treatment approach may be necessary for a successful outcome, including appropriately addressing and treating any secondary infections and breaking the itch-lick cycle. Clients may need to be advised of a guarded prognosis for complete resolution of some chronic lesions.

ACKNOWLEDGMENTS

Special thanks to Diana Loeffler, DVM, DACVP, for allowing use of the photomicrographs; to Diana Rosenberg, DVM, DACVR, for aiding in interpretation of radiographs; and to Rod Rosychuk, DVM, DACVIM, for granting permission for use of the HEET/bitter apple recipe.

REFERENCES

1. Hill PB, Lo A, Eden CA, et al. Survey of the prevalence, diagnosis and treatment of dermatological conditions in small animals in general practice. Vet Rec 2006; 158(16):533–9.

2. Yeruhum I, Gur Y, Harmelin A. Acral lick dermatitis in a dairy cow. Vet Rec 1992; 130:479–81.

3. Yeruhum I, Nyska A. Acral lick dermatitis in a jackal (*Canis aureus*). J Zoo Wildl Med 1998;29:233.

4. Kenny D. Use of naltrexone for treatment of psychogenically induced dermatoses in five zoo animals. J Am Vet Med Assoc 1994;205:1021–3.

5. Kellner CH, George MS, Burns CM, et al. Human equivalent of acral lick. Lancet 1992;339:553.

6. Shumaker AK, Angus JC, Coyner KS, et al. Microbiological and histopathological features of canine acral lick dermatitis. Vet Dermatol 2008;19:288–98.

7. Miller WH, Griffin CE, Campbell KL. Acral lick dermatitis. In: Miller WH, Griffin CE, Campbell KL, editors. Muller and Kirk's small animal dermatology. 7th edition. St Louis (MO): Elsevier; 2013. p. 650–3.

8. MacDonald J. Acral lick dermatitis. In: Bonagura JD, editor. Kirk's current veterinary therapy XV. Small animal practice. Philadelphia: WB Saunders; 2014. E-Book Chapter 33.

9. Steiss JE, Bradley DM, MacDonald J, et al. Letters to the editor. Vet Dermatol 1995;6(2):115–6.

10. Moriello K, Coyner K, Paterson S, et al. Diagnosis and treatment of dermatophytosis in dogs and cats. Vet Dermatol 2017;28(3):266-e68.

11. Goldberger E, Rapoport JL. Canine acral lick dermatitis: response to antiobsessional drug clomipramine. J Am Anim Hosp Assoc 1991;22:179–82.

12. Stein DJ, Mendelsohn I, Potocnik F, et al. Use of the serotonin reuptake inhibitor citalopram in a possible animal analogue of obsessive-compulsive disorder. Depress Anxiety 1998;8(1):39–42.

13. Wynchank D, Berk M. Fluoxetine treatment of acral lick dermatitis in dogs: a placebo-controlled randomized double blind trial. Depress Anxiety 1998;8:21–3.

14. Rapoport JL, Ryland DH, Kriete M. Drug treatment of canine acral lick. An animal model of obsessive-compulsive disorder. Arch Gen Psychiatry 1992;49:517–21.

15. Mertens P. Compulsive behavior in dogs. NAVC Clinician's Brief 2003;15–6.

16. Virga V. Behavioral dermatology. Vet Clin North Am Small Anim Pract 2003;33(2): 231–51.

17. Pereria JT, Larson CE, Ramos D, et al. Environmental, individual and triggering aspects of dogs presenting with psychogenic acral lick dermatitis [abstract]. J Vet Behav 2010;5(3):165.

18. Rosychuck RA. Canine lick granuloma. In: world small animal veterinary association world congress proceedings. 2011. Available at: https://www.vin.com/Members/proceedings. Accessed February 17, 2018.

19. Moon J, Lee P, Kim Y, et al. Efficacy and safety of 0.625% and 1.25% capsaicin patch in peripheral neuropathic pain: multi-center, randomized, and semi-double blind study. Pain Physician 2016;20:27–35.

20. Sommer C, Cruccu G. Topical treatment of peripheral neuropathic pain: applying the evidence. J Pain Symptom Manage 2017;53(3):614–29.

21. Anderson HH, Arendt-Nielson L, Elberling J. Topical capsaicin 8% for the treatment of neuropathic itch. Clin Exp Dermatol 2017;42(5):596–8.

22. Anderson HH, Marker JB, Hoeck EA, et al. Antipruritic effect of pretreatment with topical capsaicin 8% on histamine- and cowhage-evoked itch in healthy volunteers: a randomized, vehicle-controlled, proof-of-concept trial. Br J Dermatol 2017;177(1):107–16.

23. Marsella R, Nicklin CF, Melloy C. The effects of capsaicin topical therapy in dogs with atopic dermatitis: a randomized, double-blinded, placebo-controlled, cross-over clinical trial. Vet Dermatol 2002;13(3):131–9.
24. Boord M. Laser in dermatology. Clin Tech Small Anim Pract 2006;21(3):145–9.
25. Duclos D. Lasers in veterinary dermatology. Vet Clin North Am Small Anim Pract 2006;36:15–37, v.
26. Azra R. Using CO_2 laser on acral lick granulomas. Vet Pract News 2016;32–3.
27. Proshaka J, Bermudez R. Cryosurgery. StatPearls Publishing; 2018.
28. De Queiroz GF, Matera JM, Zaidan Dagli ML. Clinical study of cryosurgery efficacy in the treatment of skin and subcutaneous tumors in dogs and cats. Vet Surg 2008;37(5):438–43.
29. Biery DN. Radiation therapy in dermatology In: current veterinary therapy. WB Saunders: Philadelphia: 1968. p. 289–90.
30. Owen LN. Canine lick granuloma treated with radiotherapy. J Small Anim Pract 1989;30:454–6.
31. Budgin J, Flaherty M. Alternative therapies in veterinary dermatology. Vet Clin North Am Small Anim Pract 2013;43:189–204.
32. Lundeberg T, Bondesson L, Tomas M. Effect of acupuncture on experimentally induced itch. Br J Dermatol 1987;117(6):771–7.
33. Belgrade MJ, Solomon LM, Lichter EA. Effect of acupuncture on experimentally induced itch. Acta Derm Venereol 1984;64(2):129–33.
34. Lindley S, Cummings M. Acupuncture for the treatment of non-painful conditions. In: Lindley S, Cummings M, editors. Essentials of western veterinary acupuncture. 1st edition. Ames (IA): Blackwell Publishing; 2006. p. 129–50.
35. Pavicic Z, Potocnjac D, Krsnik B, et al. Effective use of acupuncture in treating acral lick dermatitis in a dog. Abstract. 2001. Available at: https://www.researchgate.net. Accessed March 30, 2018.
36. Paul ED, Chen A. Neural circuitry of stress, fear, and anxiety: focus on extended amygdala corticotropin-releasing factor systems. In: Fink G, editor. Stress: neuroendocrinology and neurobiology, handbook of stress, vol. 2. London: Elsevier; 2017. p. 83–96.
37. Hewson CJ, Luescher A, Parent JM, et al. Efficacy of clomipramine in the treatment of canine compulsive disorder. J Am Vet Med Assoc 1998;213(12):1760–6.
38. White S. Naltrexone for treatment of acral lick dermatitis in dogs. J Am Vet Med Assoc 1990;196(7):1073–6.
39. Dodman NH, Shuster L, Court MH, et al. Behavioral effects of narcotic antagonists. J Assoc Vet Anesthetists 1988;15:56–64.

Finish Strong.

Get a Superior USMLE Step 3 Score to Strengthen your Fellowship Applications

Step 3 CCS Bank + Question Bank:

- Be the best of the best with a superior CCS prep tool online!
- Use more than 1500 questions and 100 case simulations to get as close to the real test as possible
- Select cases by specialty, setting or topic to customize your experience
- Review question bank results by setting, problem/disease, clinical encounter, physician task, patient age

SUBSCRIBE TODAY TO SAVE 30%*

+ BONUS!

FREE Step 3 Scorrelator™ with purchase of any Question Bank to see how your scores compare to others' USMLE Step 3 and COMLEX Level III performance

NEW FRED V2 test interface for a more accurate simulation experience

---

Simple instructions to start boosting your scores:

1. Visit www.usmleconsult.com
2. Choose your Step, product and subscription length
3. Register or log in with your personal details
4. Activate discount code **CLINICS30** to calculate savings

DON'T FORGET! USMLE Consult is MAC-compatible!!

Turn to USMLE Consult for the best remediation in the business!

Elsevier is the proud publisher of USMLE Consult, Adam Brochert's Crush Step 3, and The Clinics of North America.

Activate discount code **CLINICS30** in the shopping cart to redeem savings. Offer includes all Step 3 products and all subscription lengths. Expires 12-31-2010.

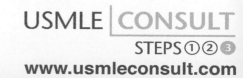

USMLE | CONSULT
STEPS ① ② ③
www.usmleconsult.com

Printed and bound by CPI Group (UK) Ltd, Croydon, CR0 4YY

13/10/2024

01773496-0001